"The deaf person—so far from being liable to be left out—is often in a strong position psychologically, like a mountain surrounded by Mahomets. Though this is only true of those who have dominated, not merely accepted, the disability. Every disability offers the same alternative: either it dominates you or you dominate it."

"One way to forget one is deaf (or blind, or a dwarf, or whatever) is to have to concentrate on making others forget it."

"Not being able to overhear, rather than not being able to hear, is the real turn of the screw. Being overheard is a related problem. For I have no judgement of how far the voice can carry, or of what noises may mask it. In crowds, or where people are about, the instinct is to lower the voice—particularly when what I have to say is not meant for the general ear. Conversely my impulse is to raise it in empty places or where no one is around. So I have an involuntary and maddening tendency to whisper at parties but shout in churches.

"The handicapped are less at the mercy of vague unhappinesses that afflict so many, especially those without aim in life, whose consequent boredom promotes what used to be called spleen. The disabled have been given a built-in, ready-packed objective which is always present: a definite impediment to get the better of. Like the prospect of hanging, it concentrates the faculties wonderfully." —*David Wright*

Deafness

ALSO BY DAVID WRIGHT

Poetry

Moral Stories
Monologue of a Deaf Man
Adam at Evening
Nerve Ends

Prose

Roy Campbell
*Algarve
*Minho and North Portugal
*with Patrick Swift

Translations

Beowulf
The Canterbury Tales

Anthologies

The Penguin Book of English Romantic Verse
The Mid-Century: English Poetry 1940-60
Longer Contemporary Poems

Deafness
David Wright

Stein and Day/*Publishers*/New York

FIRST STEIN AND DAY PAPERBACK EDITION, 1975

First published in 1969
Copyright © 1969 by David Wright
Library of Congress Catalog No. 71-87964
Printed in the United States of America
Stein and Day/*Publishers*/Scarborough House,
Briarcliff Manor, New York 10510
ISBN 0-8128-1805-9

FOR MY MOTHER AND FATHER

Mais sans changer la blanche à la noire couleur,
Et soubs nom de plaisir déguiser la douleur,
Je diray qu'estre sourd (à qui la difference
Sçait du bien & du mal) n'est mal qu'en apparence.

JOACHIM DU BELLAY

Acknowledgements

Some material of this book
has already appeared in *Encounter* and *London Magazine*.
I am indebted to C. H. Sisson
for permission to quote three lines from his poem
'My Life and Times' quoted in Chapter 1,
to Mr Kenneth W. Hodgson
for extracts from *The Deaf and their Problems*;
to Mrs Freddy Bloom
for an extract from *Our Deaf Children*;
to Leo Sherley-Price and Penguin Books for an
extract from his translation of Bede's
History of the English Church and People.

Contents

First Part

Monologue of a Deaf Man

Et lui comprit trop bien, n'ayant pas entendu.
TRISTAN CORBIÈRE

It is a good plan, and began with childhood
As my fortune discovered, only to hear
How much it is necessary to have said.
Oh silence, independent of a stopped ear,
You observe birds, flying, sing with wings instead.

Then do you console yourself? You are consoled
If you are, as all are. So easy a youth
Still unconcerned with the concern of a world
Where, masked and legible, a moment of truth
Manifests what, gagged, a tongue should have told;

Still observer of vanity and courage
And of these mirror as well; that is something
More than a sound of violin to assuage
What the human being most dies of: boredom
Which makes hedgebirds clamour in their blackthorn cage.

But did the brushless fox die of eloquence?
No, but talked himself, it seems, into a tale.
The injury, dominated, is an asset:
It is there for domination, that is all.
Else what must faith do deserted by mountains?

Talk to me then, you who have so much to say,
Spectator of the human conversation,
Reader of tongues, examiner of the eye,
And detective of clues in every action,
What could a voice, if you heard it, signify?

The tone speaks less than a twitch and a grimace.
People make to depart, do not say 'Goodbye.'
Decision, indecision, drawn on every face

As if they spoke. But what do they really say?
You are not spared, either, the banalities.

In whatever condition, whole, blind, dumb,
Onelegged or leprous, the human being is,
I affirm the human condition is the same,
The heart half broken in ashes and in lies,
But sustained by the immensity of the divine.

Thus I too must praise out of a quiet ear
The great creation to which I owe I am
My grief and my love. O hear me if I cry
Among the din of birds deaf to their acclaim,
Involved like them in the not unhearing air.

One

It is quite natural. Some hear more pleasantly
with the eyes than with the ears. I do.
GERTRUDE STEIN

ABOUT deafness I know everything and nothing. Everything, if forty years' firsthand experience is to count. Nothing, when I realize the little I have had to do with the converse aspects of deafness – the other half of the dialogue. Of that side my wife knows more than I. So do teachers of the deaf and those who work among them; not least, people involuntarily but intensely involved – ordinary men and women who find themselves, from one cause or another, parents of a deaf child. For it is the non-deaf who absorb a large part of the impact of the disability. The limitations imposed by deafness are often less noticed by its victims than by those with whom they have to do.

Deafness is a disability without pathos. Dr Johnson called it 'the most desperate of human calamities'. Yet its effects are slapstick:

'Where's the baby?'

'I put it in the dustbin.'*

There is a buffoonery about deafness which is liable to rub off on anybody who comes into contact with it. Having to shout at the hard of hearing is not elegant, nor is finger-spelling or the mouthing of words to magnify lip movements for those whose eyes are their ears. Deafness is a banana skin: an aspect which may conveniently be illustrated by an anecdote I recently came across in an old memoir. It concerns the once famous but now forgotten Victorian poet, Alexander Smith. Variations of this incident, I may add, have pursued me through life. Smith, then a young man in the early bloom of literary repute, had been taken by Swinburne's friend John Nichol to pay his respects to that formidable but deaf bluestocking, Harriet Martineau:

Miss Martineau, it is otherwise well known, is a little hard of hearing.

* To a lipreader the words *baby* and *paper* are indistinguishable.

When the travellers arrived, several ladies were with her, and by the little circle of petticoats they were received with some *empressement*. Mr Nichol took up the running, and some little conversation proceeded, Smith, in the racing phrase, *waiting*. Presently he 'came with a rush' and observed it 'had been a very fine day' – an unimpeachable and excellent remark which brought him instantly into difficulties. Miss Martineau was at once on the *qui vive*. The poet had made a remark probably instinct with fine genius, worthy of the author of *The Life Drama*. 'Would Mr Smith be so good as to repeat what he said?' Mr Smith – looking, no doubt, uncommonly like an ass – repeated it in a somewhat higher key. Alas! Alas! in vain. The old lady shook her head. 'It was really *so* annoying, but she did not quite catch it; would Mr Smith be *again* so good?' and her hand was at her eager ear. The unhappy bard, feeling, as he said, in his distress as if suicide might be the thing, shrieked and again shrieked his little piece of information – symptoms of ill-suppressed merriment becoming obvious around him. Finally the old lady's ear-trumpet was produced, and proceeding to shriek through this instrument, of which the delicate use was unknown to him, the bard nearly blew her head off.

The suffering, it will be seen, lay more to the side of Mr Smith than the deaf lady, even if she did nearly have her head blown off. Hard to bear is the devaluation of whatever one may be saying – which is almost inevitable after its fourth or fifth repetition. Yet the anecdote illustrates an undramatic but not minor disadvantage of deafness, felt less positively by the deaf than their hearing friends: having to dispense with the easy exchange of trivialities which is oil to the wheels of conversation and to the business of living. The use of language as gesture, as reassuring noise rather than an instrument of specific communication, is largely denied the deaf.

Harriet Martineau, who underwent a partial loss of hearing at the age of twenty, was one of the relatively few to write about deafness from experience. There is a surprising amount of unsentimental good sense in her *Letter to the Deaf*, bossy and dogmatic though she is. However she does put her finger on a main problem of describing deafness at first hand, when she recognizes how far the experience of it must vary from one person to another. That it must differ according to the severity of the hearing loss is obvious.

Very few are absolutely deaf. Their experience must necessarily be different from that of the severely deaf, the partially deaf, and the merely hard of hearing. The partially deaf, it seems to me, have the worst of both worlds. They hear enough to be distracted by noise yet not enough for it to be meaningful. For the merely hard of hearing there is the strain of extracting significance from sounds that may be as loud as life yet out of focus; what comes through is an auditory fuzz. Of course there are hearing-aids, but not everybody can profit from these.

Yet what is crucial is the age at which hearing is lost. Those who have been born deaf, whether completely or partially, must always be at a disadvantage compared with those who lose hearing later in life. The deaf-born cannot pick up speech and language naturally like ordinary children. They have to be taught, a difficult and slow process, the slower and more difficult the later the teaching begins. For the most intense activity of the brain takes place in the first few years of one's life, and thereafter – from the age of about three – gradually decreases. That is why small children quickly and easily pick up foreign languages while older children and adults find it an effort. But the born deaf and those who become deaf in early childhood have the compensation that they do not feel the loss of a faculty they never had or cannot remember. They are at least spared the painful effort of adjustment. The later in life one loses hearing, the sharper the test of character and fortitude: because adaptability lessens with age. On the other hand the years of hearing are so much money in the bank. Those to whom deafness comes late do not have to acquire with pain and struggle the elements of language, vocabulary, speech. These assets – pure gold – are theirs already.

It is as a deaf person that I write this book, though deafness does not seem to me to be a disproportionate element of the predicament in which I find myself; that is to say the predicament in which we are all involved because we live and breathe. If vocation means anything, I suppose myself a poet. Whether I am that is disputable, but the deafness remains a fact.

I propose, then, to begin with my own firsthand experience of the nature and effects of deafness – it is what I know about. But also

> Because 'I am' may read 'We are'.
> Remember that the human race
> Grins, more or less, from every face.

None the less the reader must bear very much in mind that the experience of deafness varies according to its type, the age at which it is contracted, the disposition, temperament, and predilections of the individual. My own experience of deafness must have been different had I been even a few years older or younger when I lost my hearing. It must also have been different had I wanted to be an engineer or a farmer instead of a poet.* But in each case in detail only, for the basic situation would have been the same. And in this sense to experience a particular disability like deafness is to share a common experience with all who have been disabled. As a deaf man I feel *en rapport* with other kinds of cripples, whether blind, spastic, legless, etc.; and they with me, unless I deceive myself. It's not that cripples are sympathetic to cripples, far from it. But they share a firsthand knowledge of disablement. They can and do see one another objectively – a lame duck doesn't have to feel sorry for a lame duck. The cataract of pity does not cloud the field of vision.

So far as cripples are concerned pity is no virtue. It is a sentiment that deceives its bestower and disparages its recipient. Helen Keller hated it, and she was blind as well as deaf. Its acceptance not only humiliates, but actually blunts the tools needed to best the disability. To accept pity means taking the first step towards self-pity, thence to the finding, and finally the manufacture, of excuses. The end-product of self-exculpation is the failed human being, the victim. As the cliché runs – 'victim of circumstances beyond his control' – as if anybody were in control of circumstances. But one should draw a distinction between pity and compassion. Compassion springs from charity (we could use the word love, were it not devalued). Pity is the coin Dives threw at Lazarus: 'Take this, it shows I have more money (or whatever) than you'; compassion is the kind of concern expressed by the good Samaritan ('I might be in your case') who interrupted his journey and put himself out to help the other. Compassion is hard. It makes a moral and intellectual demand; it is not concerned with the ego.

Now I must emphasize that I am completely without hearing – a fact, so rum is the operation of human vanity, on which I rather pique myself. (When introducing me to people my mother

---

*Deaf poets are not quite as rare as blind painters, though perhaps they ought to be. Two of the greatest poets of the renaissance, Pierre de Ronsard and Joachim du Bellay, were deaf from early youth. Du Bellay addressed a *Hymne à la Surdité* to Ronsard. Among living poets there is Jack Clemo, who is both blind and deaf.

still says, 'He's a little deaf' – a euphemism I find vaguely defamatory.) Total deafness is comparatively rare, which may be an advantage from the point of view of this book – such a degree of deafness may serve as a criterion.

I do not live in a world of complete silence. There is no such thing as absolute deafness. Coming from one whose aural nerve is extinct, this statement may be taken as authoritative.

Let me attempt to define the auditory limits of the world I inhabit. They are perhaps less restricted than may be imagined. Without entering into technicalities about sones, decibels, and so on, it may be said that all sound is vibration and that the ear, roughly speaking, is a highly specialized organ for the reception of air-vibrations or sound-waves. But other things beside air conduct vibration and therefore sound – wood for instance. If I stand on a wooden floor I can 'hear' footsteps behind me, but not when standing on a floor made of some less resonant substance – for example stone or concrete. I can even partially 'hear' my own voice. This is not surprising, for people hear themselves talk mainly by bone-conduction inside their heads (but other persons by air-conduction; that is why people find their own voices sounding surprisingly different when thrown back at them by a tape recorder). Yet like nearly all deaf people I cannot judge the loudness or quality of my own voice. To some extent I can do so by putting a finger against my Adam's apple or voicebox. This is well known as one of the ways in which the deaf can be made to 'hear' something of a speech-instructor's voice. Likewise I 'hear' a piano if I place a finger on it while it is being played; a radio and gramophone too, when touching the sound box or amplifier. (The gramophone needle gives best results, but this isn't good for the record.) Such 'hearing' is selective; I receive only the low notes of the scale, the high ones elude me. No matter how loud the volume is turned on what comes through is a bent or incomplete version of actual sound. In 'touch-hearing' most music, and all speech, comes across as a blurry bumble of noise.

Nevertheless there is some music that I enjoy after a fashion. But it has to be produced by stringed instruments (harp, guitar, piano, double-bass, and so on) as I cannot hear wind-instruments (flute, bagpipes, oboe). Percussive instruments like drums are naturally well inside my range. I have a passion for military bands, though hearing little except the drumtaps, a sad boom-thud from the big drum and a clattering exhilaration from the kettledrums. But I can't recognize a tune, not even 'God Save the Queen'. Since I lost my hearing there is only one musical work of which I can lay my hand on my heart and say it has truly given me an aesthetic experience. This is Bach's Italian Concerto. When I was an undergraduate at Oxford a German friend of mine often played it on the piano. The piece bewitched me. Luckily it was one of his favourites for I used to make him play the concerto over and over again. Perhaps rather highbrow a bit of music to get a fixation on. Yet when he tried me out with Beethoven, Mozart, Mendelssohn, and even other pieces by Bach, I got nothing. Later I 'listened' to Sibelius, Britten, Stravinsky and so forth – to all sorts of music, folk, pop, and concrete – but none of them meant a thing.

Though it is nearly a quarter of a century since I heard it played, the Italian Concerto remains part of my spiritual furniture. Not long ago I tried to reproduce what I could remember of it, or rather of its effect upon myself, in the course of a poem. I offer the verses here for their interest as attempted onomatopoeic re-creation of piano music as heard, so to speak, by deaf ears:

PIANO

Openhanded, opionated, cracked, she lived alone
Survivor of ordinary sorrows: which to assuage
Death, being no enemy, subtracted her from knowledge.
She is now and forever absent from her music-room
Unless as an essence contained in its weatherwarped thin
Panellings impregnated with the repeated passage
And phrasing of Beethoven, Brahms. Their reverberate message
She would draw from a grand piano, plundering from the strung

Harp hidden within, cunningly manipulating
The obedience of keys as some Dresden musician taught her –
Flood and ebb of sonata over an empty lawn
Clear of a ratiocination of grief – rapt in her
Artificial beatitude, world constructed of sound,
The articulate mathematical order of which we are given an
    inkling.

To get on with the list of things audible, or at least interfering with the silence that might be expected to compensate a totally occluded ear, let me tabulate the following: gunfire, detonation of high-explosive, low-flying aeroplanes, cars backfiring, motor-bicycles, heavy lorries, carts clattering over cobblestones, wurlitzers, pneumatic drills. There can't be much that I miss of the normal orchestration of urban existence. I should add that I also, once, heard the human voice. One day in 1963 I was at Lord's cricket ground; Ted Dexter had just come in to bat against the West Indies. He put a couple of runs on the board with the air of a man who means to get another ninety-eight before lunch. Suddenly he was bowled. While the bails were still flying, coats, hats, cushions, umbrellas, sandwiches, for all I know babies even, were hurled into the air by some nine or ten thousand West Indians in the free seats where I was watching. Up went a simultaneous roar of delight. Hearing that sound, for me not very loud but like a croaking bark, was a queer and spooky experience. I have never forgotten it.

It will be seen that the world a deaf man inhabits is not one of complete silence, which is perhaps the chief complaint he has to make about it. There is another point. Though noise, as such, does not obtrude to the extent that the above catalogue would seem to imply, the world in which I live seldom *appears* silent. Let me try to explain what I mean. In my case, silence is not absence of sound but of movement.

Suppose it is a calm day, absolutely still, not a twig or leaf stirring. To me it will seem quiet as a tomb though hedgerows are full of noisy but invisible birds. Then comes a breath of air, enough to unsettle a leaf; I will see and hear that movement like an exclamation. The illusory soundlessness has been interrupted. I see, as if I heard, a visionary noise of wind in a disturbance of foliage. Wordsworth in a late poem exactly caught the phenomenon in a remarkable line:

A soft eye-music of slow-waving boughs

which may have subconsciously derived from an equally cogent line in Coleridge's *The Eolian Harp*:

A light in sound, a sound-like power of light.

The 'sound' seen by me is not necessarily equivalent to the real one. It must often be close enough, in my case helped by a subliminal memory of things once heard. I cannot watch a gale without 'hearing' an uproar of violent movement: trees thrashing, grassblades battling and flattened; or, at sea, waves locked and staggering like all-in wrestlers – this kind of thing comes through as hubbub enough. On the other hand I also live in a world of sounds which are, as I know quite well, imaginary because non-existent. Yet for me they are part of reality. I have sometimes to make a deliberate effort to remember I am not 'hearing' anything, because there is nothing to hear. Such non-sounds include the flight and movement of birds, even fish swimming in clear water or the tank of an aquarium. I take it that the flight of most birds, at least at a distance, must be silent – bar the creaking noise made by the wings of swans and some kinds of wild geese. Yet it *appears* audible, each species creating a different 'eye-music', from the nonchalant melancholy of seagulls to the staccato flitting of tits.

This is not to subscribe to the irritating theory that the loss of one sense is compensated for by the quickening of another. There are no compensations, life is not like that. At best we are offered alternatives. We have no choice but to take them.

This is by no means a complete picture of the world I live in, or of any other deaf person's, come to that. Almost nothing has been said about the major hurdle of deafness, the problem of communication. It is simply an attempt to convey what deafness is like physically, or at least what it's like so far as one deaf man is concerned, before I go on to tell the story of how I lost my hearing, how I reacted, how I was educated, and the various stratagems necessity forced me to adopt to get on and get by in a non-deaf world.

For I am now, after forty years of what we will term silence, so accommodated to it (like a hermit-crab to its shell) that were the faculty of hearing restored to me tomorrow it would appear an affliction rather than a benefit. I do not mean that I find deafness desirable but that in the course of time the disability has been assimilated to the extent that it is now an integral condition of existence, like the use of a hand. By the same token the restoration of my hearing, or the loss of my deafness, whichever is the right way of putting it, would be like having that hand cut off.

Two

The first thing that strikes me
on hearing a Misfortune having befallen another is this:
'Well it cannot be helped – he will have the pleasure of
trying the resources of his spirit.'

JOHN KEATS

UP to the age of seven I was exceptionally lucky, or – which is
the same thing – happy in my childhood.

My parents were well off. We lived in a house with a large
garden. If I had no brothers or sisters I had them ready-made, so
to speak, in the children of the neighbours. Our house was one of
five others, each standing in its own ground and built on the side
of a kopje* which overlooks Orange Grove, then an outlying
suburb of Johannesburg. They commanded a panorama of the
high veld: a plateau rolling towards the blue indentations of the
Magaliesberg forty miles to the north. The kopje above and behind our houses was still virgin bush, not altogether abandoned
by its aboriginal fauna – mostly rock-rabbits and snakes; there
were also lizards and chameleons. Insect-life was more spectacular – praying-mantises, millipedes, beetles and armoured scor-
pions, an occasional storm of locusts; and in summer, unbelievable clouds of butterflies of every size and colour, more brilliant
than the flowers they fed on. Birds of all kinds, whose names I
never learned (except for European visitors like the swallows)
inhabited the air; in particular a species of goldfinch that wove
globular nests of grass which, suspended by a few plaited wisps
from the branches of a tree, looked exactly like the coloured glass
balls used for Christmas decorations. There was even game: as
late as 1930 I would often come across the spoor of duiker – a
kind of small buck – in the eucalyptus plantations a mile or two
from our house.

That environment has mostly disappeared. The open veld beyond Louis Botha Avenue has of course been built over; and the

* Small hill.

great green and golden mimosas which once embowered the old Orange Grove Hotel have long been chopped down. The Orange Grove Hotel had stood for perhaps a quarter of a century and was one of the oldest buildings in the neighbourhood; for Johannesburg did not exist, nor was the gold of Witwatersrand so much as a prospector's myth, when my mother was born. Yet Johannesburg seemed to my childhood eye to be of immeasurable antiquity. In those days I would have been incredulous to learn that Graaff's, the Greek shop at the corner of Louis Botha Avenue, had not existed from the beginning of time.

Johannesburg in the early nineteen-twenties was a town of concrete office-blocks, bungalows, red corrugated-iron roofs; of trams and dust; of high-slung brass-lanterned motor-cars competing with long, magnificent oxwagon trains – each drawn by eight span or more of extravagantly horned oxen – which were still a major form of transport in South Africa. The skyscrapers, the glass palaces, the flats like cubic boxes, the megalomaniac suburban villas, were yet to be built. But it was necklaced by a circle of white mine-dumps floating like gulls on the wide ocean of the high veld: they are still, perhaps, the only purely beautiful constructs of the whole city.*

In our suburb we had the advantage of living in both town and country. For at least six months of the year we never slept under a roof, but on the stoep† in the open. This was in winter. Our winters were bone-dry – the days baking hot and the nights, because of the altitude, colder than needles. I used to wake in the mornings to find the glass of water at my bedside frozen solid. My ceiling was the night sky, and became my entertainment; some of the constellations – the sword and belt of Orion – I learned to recognize before I knew what they were or that they had names. In summer we slept indoors, for summer was the rainy season.

The pattern of our weather hardly ever varied. As a rule a summer morning led off with a cloudless sky. But about eleven o'clock huge bales of cumuli would begin to create themselves, rather like Hoyle's hydrogen atoms appearing in space from nowhere. These clouds would clap on sail, skysails over their royals, close with one another and grapple, till by around 3 p.m. nothing would be visible but their garboard strakes overlaying the entire heaven.

---

*I am told they are now being done away with.
† Verandah.

14

At four in the afternoon (you could almost set your watch by it) there would be a moment of intense quiet, then a brief chill gust of wind. As if that were a signal of battle, the cloud-car-racks overhead would loose off a simultaneous broadside: an earsplitting barrage whose reverberations seemed to rumble on to the extremities of the visible world until the next appalling uproar of thunder drowned the penultimate echoes of the last. Then the clouds would split like burst flourbags, discharging solid bolts of rain. A really bad thunderstorm might contribute bounc-ing bullets of hail, some as big as golfballs and guaranteed to flatten a garden or lay waste an orchard.

Most English-speaking South Africans are either recent arrivals, or descendants of the Uitlanders who came to make their for-tunes in the Kimberley diamond-fields or the Transvaal gold-mines. My father came of older stock; his family went back to the 1820 Settlers, the first British emigrants to South Africa. A con-sequence of the Napoleonic Wars had been economic distress in England. One of the ideas for relieving this had been the estab-lishment of a settlement in the new and apparently useless Cape Colony which Britain had annexed in the course of the struggle. The 1820 Settlers of Albany, a district near Port Elizabeth, were the result. Another object of the scheme, one that was probably glossed over in the prospectus for would-be emigrants, was to plant a sort of buffer-state – a defence-in-depth of colonists with a stake in the land – between the more or less nomadic Boer farmers of Cape Colony and the Xhosa tribesmen, their cattle-raiding neighbours on the other side of the Fish River. Like all pioneers the 1820 Settlers had a rough deal. Besides having to attend to problems presented by the weather and local wild life (lions, leopards, hippopotami), most of the later Kaffir Wars were fought over their territory. Instead of being welcome allies, the Settlers seem to have been a final feather in the balance so far as the Boers were concerned. Not long after their appearance the Boers decided to turn their backs, not so much on the British as on Europe itself, and in 1836 began their Great Trek into the wilder-ness, out of reach of evangelical missionaries and nineteenth-century progressiveness – out of reach, too, of more admirable manifestations of the European zeitgeist – where they have stayed ever since. As for the Settlers, most of them eventually abandoned their farms and took up urban employment, for which they were really better suited. And since then, as someone has pointed out, the English South Africans have tended to live in towns and Afrikaners (as the Boers are now called) in the country.

My father was descended on both sides from these colonists. Only one of his forebears seems ever to have achieved distinction. This was a Captain Manley from Yorkshire, who served in the Kaffir Wars as A.D.C. to Sir Harry Smith.* The Captain is said to have been responsible for improving the climate of Grahamstown, which used to be notably arid even by South African standards. Apparently the Captain, ahead of such bright notions, concluded that if trees could be induced to grow there they might attract moisture. He guessed that Australian wattle and blue gum would do the trick, planted the trees, and bingo! down came the rain. So runs family tradition, in proof of which I am told that a tract of land near Grahamstown is to this day called Manley's Flats.

One of the Captain's daughters married my grandfather, Ormson David Wright, of whose life I wish I knew more. All I know of him is that when the diamond-fields were discovered in 1870 he trekked four hundred miles to Kimberley as a boy of fourteen, trudging behind his stepfather's oxwagon while his mother followed in a buggy. There he made a fortune in diamonds, sold out to Barney Barnato† and turned to the Stock Exchange. Here he made another fortune which he managed to lose just before the Boer War. Apparently he left a partner in charge of his stockbroking business while he made the grand tour of Europe. The partner absconded. So my grandfather came back to South Africa and started all over again; this time in Johannesburg, where he soon repaired his bank balance. This fortune he was also to mislay partly owing to the 1929 stock market crash and partly because

---

*Sir Harry Smith (1787–1860), still a legendary figure in South Africa but half-forgotten in England, like so many nineteenth-century heroes who had fabulous but peripheral careers. He fought in almost every battle of the Peninsular War, was at Waterloo, and even managed to be present at the burning of the Capitol in Washington. He married a Spanish girl whom he rescued at the sack of Badajoz. She became almost as legendary as himself (two South African towns, Harrismith and Ladysmith, are named after them). Harry Smith was the hero of the famous Ride to the relief of Grahamstown during the Kaffir Wars – six hundred miles in six days. He interrupted his South African career to become victor of the battle of Aliwal in the Sikh War; and closed it as Governor of Cape Colony.

† The Cockney millionaire to whom Cecil Rhodes made out the famous £5,000,000 cheque that gave him control of the diamond industry.

his confidential clerk embezzled scrip (he seems to have had no luck with business partners). A few years after the crash my grandfather died almost penniless in the bedsitting-room of a suburban boarding-house.

I remember him well, in the days both of his magnificence – the chauffeured limousine, Rand Club and Members' Pavilion at the Wanderers (he had played cricket against Lord Hawke's team in the eighties) – and of his hard-up old age. Rich or broke, he always looked as immaculate as if he had stepped out of a bandbox. To the day of his death he was known as 'the best-dressed man in South Africa'. Poverty must have been hard to meet after his kind of life, but he never gave it the satisfaction of hearing him grumble.

But in 1927 the stock market was booming. My father was a partner in my grandfather's stockbroking firm. I was seven years old and had just begun attending St John's Preparatory School on the outskirts of Houghton Estate. St John's was a High Anglican sort of place. The headmaster was a priest – Father Something-or-other; I remember him but not his name. After all, I only attended the school for a single term.

This was to be my sole experience – apart from a kindergarten at Hope Road where I had been taught to read, write, and count – of 'normal' education. I was assigned to a classroom where a pretty young woman taught, or at least kept under control, some twenty or thirty little boys of my own age. Her lessons, or some of them, I remember vividly, perhaps because they are among my last aural memories. She used to read poetry to us – probably to keep us quiet. This was mostly A. A. Milne's children's verse, which I liked, though it dealt with a strange world of white nannies and gardeners, of flora and fauna and of seasons that seemed to bear no relation to the one we lived in. We had chapel on Thursday mornings; one of the fathers used to preach excellent little sermons. Plenty of incense and candles, organ-music and hymn-singing.

> There is a green hill far away
> Without a city wall ...

I used to worry about that green hill having no city wall; it never occurred to me that 'without' meant 'outside'. During the morning and lunchtime breaks I was initiated into the tribalism of small boys: the rigid ritual attending games of marbles and conkers; the even more rigid taboo on playing any of those out of season; the pecking, or rather the kicking, order among contemporaries; the exhibition of penises behind the bicycle-sheds; and the acquisition, for tribal use only, of a new and arcane vocabulary.

After that one term at St John's there followed a family holiday by the sea, at a place called Plettenberg's Bay near Knysna in Cape Province. Part of the aboriginal forest there is called 'The Garden of Eden'. I took the name literally. When the hired car stopped beside a glade through which ran a stream embowered by gigantic trees and giant ferns, and the driver announced 'This is the Garden of Eden', I believed, without much inquiring as to the whereabouts of guardian angels with burning swords, that I was looking at the exact spot where our first parents had talked with alpha and omega. Even today I'm not sure I wasn't right – places and things are as sacred as we make them.

At Plettenberg's Bay we stayed at an old hotel standing on a tidal island. There was no village, no bungalows or houses or even bathing-huts, just the one building overlooking a crescent bay. My father spent most of his time fishing from the cliffs for mussel-grinders – the kind of big fish one associates with photographs of Hemingway – but seldom made a catch. Too much sun, he would say. Or too much wind. Or not enough sun or not enough wind. He might return without fish but never without a reason. Sometimes he would join us on the beach, hopping across the sand on one leg (he had lost a foot in the war) to dive in among the breakers and regain, in tumbling buoyant water, physical equality with the rest of us. Being minus a foot made no difference when swimming or surfing. *Et ego in Arcadia*. That time and place is part of the immortal present in my mind, and will be till I turn it all in. Things were to be very different soon, but that experience of felicity has paid, and still pays, for everything that later befell.

Soon after we returned to Johannesburg I contracted scarlet fever, which in 1927 was a dangerous disease. How long I lay ill I cannot tell, but it seemed to me I kept my bed for weeks, getting a little worse each day. The crisis of my illness I remember well enough. On that day I was in fact dying, though I didn't know it.

In the afternoon my father came into the room.

'Would you like me to read to you, John?'

'Yes.'

I was called John then; later, as will be seen, I changed my name. My father read very well, he had a good voice. It was not often he read to me. I felt drowsy and pleased, listening to his baritone and following the story while the afternoon sunlight altered from gold to bronze.

'Can you hear me now, John?' Every few minutes he would interrupt himself to ask that question. Of course I could hear him, I could hear him perfectly. Then I went to sleep.

That evening a *deus ex machina* arrived. The family doctor had all along taken an over-optimistic view of my case. He had refused to believe there was any danger of complications setting in until it became obvious that they had. Now it was nearly too late. The *deus ex machina*, summoned over the family doctor's head, was a Eurasian specialist of the name of Campbell. He represented my last hope. I have since thought it extraordinary that a Eurasian should have been practising as a doctor in Johannesburg. Even in those days the colour bar was not noticeably flexible, however rigid it may have since become. It was lucky for me that Dr Campbell was not debarred from treating Europeans; or I might now be dead.

Dr Campbell decided to operate on the spot. I remember his knives and instruments glittering on the dressing-table under an ornate lampshade. Except for that puddle of light the room was dark. Then the chloroform put me out.

I opened my eyes to find myself wrapped up in an eiderdown, borne in the arms of our houseboy. He was a black Zeus who had been given the working-name of Charlie. Before I fell ill he had been teaching me Zulu, of which all that remains to me now is the one phrase – *Hamba yega*! I must have heard it often enough when I came bothering him at his work. The meaning is *voetsak*, get out. Together we were descending the cold stone staircase. I caught a glimpse of my mother.

'Where are we going?' I could just see her face. She said something I didn't quite catch. The Zulu carried me out of the house into the garden, past the cedar-tree where the chameleon lived, down the zigzag stone terraces and into a black avenue of firs whose branches interlocked above our heads. When we came out of it the sky seemed full of stars. On the tarmac road a car stood waiting. Charlie deposited me in its front seat. Dr Campbell got in beside the steering-wheel. A smell of petrol floated up from the floorboards. I heard the engine start, the gears engage.

It was a hospital to which I was taken. My mother spent the night beside my bed, but in what frame of mind she kept the useless vigil – for I slept soundly – I do not care to imagine.

She was not South African but pure Scots. Like most of her family my mother had married late – indeed, her father had been born in the reign of George IV.

I have seen the birthplace of this Scottish grandfather: four stone walls, the remains of what was once a cottage and is now a sheepfold on the banks of the river Stinchar in Ayrshire. His family were highlanders from Perthshire who emigrated after the break-up of the clan system that followed the defeat of Culloden Cousins of his had been neighbours of the Burns family at Alloway near Ayr. Family legend says that as a boy one of them 'held the plough' for Robert Burns. My grandfather's name was John Murray. He was the son of a stonemason who began life as coachman to the Earl of Cassilis at Culzean Castle, and married his cook, one Margaret Bone, who is said to have been of French extraction. Himself a stonemason to begin with, my grandfather launched out as a builder. A fair bit of nineteenth-century Glasgow appears to have been built by him, as well as a number of bridges in the industrial part of Cumberland. In those days the navvies of Cumberland were a tough lot; he used to tell my mother how on pay-day he sat at a table handing out the wages with a loaded revolver in front of him. That must have been in the eighteen-sixties. His biggest job was the building of Loch Inch Castle, seat of the Earl of Stair – one of those brobdignagian Scottish baronial exercises in baroque gothic, which have to be seen to be believed. Later my grandfather took a lease of the Corsehill Quarries near Annan in Dumfriesshire. These produced a red sandstone once much used for building. At one time, before McKinley clapped a tariff on it, my grandfather made a great deal of money selling the stone to America. He even built and owned a sailing-vessel, the *Margaret Murray*, which carried cargoes to Brazil and round the Horn to Valparaiso. Her ballast of Corsehill stone was sold in the ports where she touched: much of it now forms the base of the Statue of Liberty outside New York Harbour.

It was at Annan that my mother was brought up. She was educated at its famous Academy, where Edward Irving the apoca-

lyptic preacher and his friend Thomas Carlyle had been pupils.*
But as she grew up my mother found the provincialism of the
little Border town stifling. Desperate and determined to get away
from the place, she took up one of the few careers open to
women in Edwardian days and trained as a nursing sister at Guy's
Hospital in London.

This was before the Kaiser's war. Later she would talk nostal-
gically about those London years before the knocking on the gate
in 1914. On Sunday she would go to one of the city churches, not
so much to worship as to listen to the sermon, and not so much
to listen to the sermon as to listen to the preacher's pronunciation of English. London she knew at many levels, from the slums
of the Borough, where she was on call to act at confinements
during her training as a midwife, to bohemian Soho, where the
painter Henry Lamb (who had been one of her patients) used to
take her out to dinner. In those days you could get a roast chicken
and a bottle of wine for half a crown. She seems to have attended
what must have been Edith Sitwell's first poetry reading; and she
remembers seeing the still-unfinished portrait of Lytton Strachey
in Henry Lamb's studio.

Among other things the Kaiser's war brought my father to England. He had served in the South African Rebellion and in General
Botha's short desert campaign in German West Africa. Invalided
out of his South African regiment, he sailed to England, re-
enlisted with the Royal Artillery and fought at Passchendaele. In
the end he lost a foot, but through no malice of the enemy. Riding
a motor-bicycle with faulty brakes, my father coincided with a
goods-engine at a level-crossing somewhere in France. The engine
crushed his foot and he was shipped back to England to have it
amputated. Thus he found himself at Guy's Hospital, where he
met my mother. They married in 1919, when my father took her
back with him to South Africa. The following year I was born.

My mother stayed all night by my bed in the nursing-home to
which I had been taken. But when I opened my eyes the next
morning she had gone. No sooner was I awake than I received my

---

*According to local tradition which my mother passed on to me, in
infancy Carlyle was thought to be a 'natural'. Until he was five years old he
never spoke. Then, so runs the story, in the kitchen-parlour of his home
where a new baby lay crying in its cradle, young Thomas Carlyle electrified
his parents by speaking a complete sentence 'What ails wee Jock?'

first visitor. It was my father, looking in on his way to the office.

His visit inaugurated a ceremony which was to be observed every morning so long as I stayed at the nursing-home. Pulling his gold watch (it had rococo Victorian initials engraven on the back) from his waistcoat-pocket, he would hold it up to my ear.

'Can you hear the tick?' I would shake my head. My head was thick with bandages.

My father never failed to pay his early morning visit or to administer the ritual of the watch. It gave me a first clue to the discovery I was to make in the course of the next few weeks: that I had completely lost my hearing.

One would think that deafness must have been self-evident from the first. On the contrary it took me some time to find out what had happened. I had to deduce the fact of deafness through a process of reasoning. I did not notice it. No one inhabits a world of total silence: I had 'heard' the doctor's car driving me to the hospital, while the tread of the nurse coming into my room used to wake me in the morning – how was I to know? Nobody told me.

It was made more difficult to perceive because from the very first my eyes had unconsciously begun to translate motion into sound. My mother spent most of the day beside me and I understood everything she said. Why not? Without knowing it I had been reading her mouth all my life. When she spoke I seemed to hear her voice. It was an illusion which persisted even after I knew it was an illusion. My father, my cousin, everyone I had known, retained phantasmal voices. That they were imaginary, the projections of habit and memory, did not come home to me until I had left hospital. One day I was talking with my cousin and he, in a moment of inspiration, covered his mouth with his hand as he spoke. Silence! Once and for all I understood that when I could not see I could not hear.

But that was later. Only little by little did I attain right knowledge of my condition. The watch business put me on the track. From discovering that there were some things I could not hear I progressed to the truth that I could hear nothing.

The discovery in no way upset me. It was very gradually that I understood what had happened. Then, being innocent of experience, I was spared – as my parents certainly were not spared – speculation or foresight of the ways in which the rest of my life might be modified and hampered. For my parents what had happened was a catastrophe; to me it was an incident. It seemed neither important nor extraordinary except in so far that everything seems important and extraordinary when one is seven. Like animals, children are able to accept injuries in a casual manner, with apparent courage.

Children have a resilience and adaptability that must seem unbelievable to an adult. No courage bore me up at the age of seven; nature, or whatever you call the almost unthwartable energy of life which inhabits all young creatures – the drive to go on living under any circumstances – made deafness seem to me, at the time, one of the normal accidents of living.

In the case of a deaf child it is the parents who do the suffering, at least to begin with. Mine found themselves faced with all sorts of questions to which they had to find answers that might not, for all they knew, exist. How was I to be educated? How far would I be able to lead a 'normal' life? When I grew up, would I be capable of ordinary social intercourse? How would I earn a living? You can imagine what forebodings weighed on them. They could not know that things might work out better than they feared.

It was easier for me than for those about me to accept the fact of my deafness. How should they know I was scarcely bothered by it? In the nursing-home and during my convalescence they were continually assuring me that my hearing would come back. That I might not have been very interested one way or another, none of them guessed. I had no sense of loss. I didn't mind not hearing. Not at all! But I did begin to find it exasperating to be offered, like a never-arriving birthday treat, the prospect of some magical restoration of hearing – next week, next month, next year. Promises made in all good faith: the doctors would have proffered vague hopes. Such hopes would be handed on, transmuted to near-certainties, perhaps with the idea of keeping up my spirits. No one supposed that my spirits might have no need of being kept up – I was not in pain, I was having a jolly good time at the nursing-home. But because they were repeated so often, I at first believed the rumours and prophecies of a return of hearing. After some months, when nothing had happened, I decided that the state of suspended expectation entailed by belief in these foretellings was a nuisance. Privately and deliberately I made up my mind that no matter what anybody told me I should always be deaf.

I remember coming to this conclusion, or was it resolve, one morning as I lay in bed at the nursing-home. I did not speak about it to anyone for I guessed that I would only upset people and make trouble were I to let them know what was in my mind.

Looking back, I see that this resolution was positive and not negative. From that moment I must have begun adapting to my altered prospects in life.

Three

Words are only motion and form.

FRANCIS BACON

MY becoming deaf when I did – if deafness had to be my destiny – was remarkably lucky. By the age of seven a child will have grasped the essentials of language, as I had. Having learned naturally how to speak was another advantage – pronunciation, syntax, inflection, idiom, all had come by ear. I had the basis of a vocabulary which could easily be extended by reading. All these would have been denied me had I been born deaf or lost my hearing earlier than I did. Lastly I was too young to be disorientated or emotionally incommoded by the loss, while still young enough to adapt to the disability without effort. Had deafness happened a few years later, say at the age of fourteen or twenty, I should have thought it a calamity (which it would have been) and I do not see how I should have escaped feeling very sorry for myself. Of course I did very often feel very sorry for myself, but that was long afterwards and a by-effect of puberty.

When I left the nursing-home it was for a long convalescence, chiefly spent, so far as I remember, in regaining the use of my legs. After spending months in bed I had to learn to walk all over again. No sooner was I mobile than it became necessary to undergo a second, more serious, operation to remove the mastoid bones behind my ears. This it seems was an essential follow-up to the emergency surgery performed by Dr Campbell. The operation was to be done at Cape Town. They did not tell me about it at the time of course – no point in worrying a child. So far as I was concerned we were going to the Cape for a holiday; after which, they said, I would be going to hospital to have my tonsils out.

We stayed at the home of some friends of my father's, at an old Dutch colonial farmhouse, one of the most beautiful places I ever lived in. This many-gabled limewashed mansion stood at the end of a long avenue of rheumatoid oak trees which were reputed to have been planted a hundred years before. By

Johannesburg standards all this represented almost measureless antiquity. Perhaps as a consequence it was here that I began research into the origins of the visible world. A child's version of the Bible came into my hands. Its account of the creation I found imaginatively satisfactory, as, give or take a few points of detail, I still do.

Then I was taken to a hospital standing on the lower slopes of Table Mountain. From my bed I could see the granite tooth of Devil's Peak, centrepiece of a dramatic panorama. Somehow I guessed I was in for something worse than a tonsillectomy. When they wheeled me into the operating theatre I did not at all care for the look of the surgical scissors and saws prepared for the occasion. A chloroform mask was clamped over my face.

They were right about my tonsils. Although it was the mastoid bones behind my ears that the surgeon had been after, for good measure he threw in, or threw out, my tonsils. When I came to what hurt was not my head but my throat.

Another long convalescence: this was the most boring period of my life. With my mother I stayed at a boarding-house at St James, a seaside resort near Kalk Bay, not far from Cape Town. The weather was generally rotten. It was out of season; I soon tired of walking along wintry beaches interrupted with seaweed-stinking rocks. The other diversion was to sit in the wickerwork chairs of the boarding-house lounge and look through old copies of the *Tatler* and yellow-bound weekly numbers of the *Daily Mirror* that came by sea mail, never less than a fortnight out of date. I soon found a more interesting employment in the inspection of a near-by cemetery. This I preferred to the desolation of the beach, the stifled aspidistras of the boarding-house lounge. My absorption in the cemetery worried my mother. She thought it morbid. But it was the sculptured gravestones and monuments – standard cemetery chisellings, mediocre enough no doubt – that caught my fancy. I particularly admired the effigy of a young woman with wings and a nightdress pointing an index finger at the sky. It may have been the last straw when I said to my mother:

'When I'm dead, promise me that I can have an angel on my grave.'

But it was all an embryonic feeling for sculpture; all that time a cemetery was the nearest thing to an art gallery that I had seen.

On the whole I was becoming rather impossible. Until the scarlet fever interrupted our lives my parents had treated me like an ordinary child. Now I was pitied and a focus for irrational feelings of guilt, as if they felt somehow responsible for the deafness. Naturally though not admirably I began to exploit the new attitude and trade on sympathy. Allowances were to be made? I took them. Such natural sympathy and grief-stricken understandable spoiling is a hazard encountered by most deaf children. And for the time being I was without the corrective influence of companions of my own age – all my childhood friends were in Johannesburg. It was term-time; no other children were staying at the boarding-house. I began to read a lot. My imagination fed on Hugh Lofting and comics like *The Rainbow*. I began making up interminable stories, adventures in which I figured along with the characters from whatever tale or book occupied my thoughts. These I would recount in the form of a long monologue whenever I could get my mother (a captive and appalled audience) to listen. At this period I must have been a bit odd. One specialist who examined me about then came to the conclusion that I had a screw loose. No, he did not tell my parents that – I heard it many years later from a friend of the specialist's.

At that time – it was the year before the great stock market crash – the family fortunes were at their zenith. If for myself I had accepted the conviction that deafness would be permanent, my parents had not. They still hoped. They were able, moreover, to pay for the best advice. So my mother took me to England to do a round of the specialists.

I had been to England before, when I was five, on the way to spend a few summer weeks in Scotland with my grandmother and cousins (incidentally I picked up a broad Scots accent – an acquisition that gave something less than unadulterated satisfaction to my mother, who had taken some trouble to shed hers).

This time we stayed in London, at a flat on the top floor of a house in Devonshire Terrace, on the Bayswater fringe of Paddington. We shared this flat with my mother's sister Mat and my cousin Fergus. It must have been the early autumn of 1928 when we arrived in England. We remained there till the spring or summer of 1929. For I remember the hard winter of 1928–9, skating on the Serpentine and sliding on the Round Pond. I remember, too, going for daily walks with Fergus across the park to Buckingham Palace to read the bulletins of the king's health posted on the railings. What a London that was, most of it now gone. Gaslit streets, stone pavements, neoclassical Victorian porticos, gloom and cosiness; iron trams, open-top double-decker buses, square squat taxicabs, horsedrawn vans and brewers' drays; inhabited by subfusc troglodytes, bowler-hatted or cloth-capped; a megalopolis inhibited by iron railings – park-railings, palace-railings, garden-railings, square-railings, churchyard-railings, hospital-railings, area-railings; secure; impenetrable; smug.

I did not like England. A small, sooty, crimped island beginning with plutonian railway labyrinths (we had disembarked at Liverpool) that continued under a lowering pall of bruised cloud – a constipated landscape squared off into pocket-handkerchief fields and paddocks, no open country (or what I considered open country) to be seen anywhere – that ended in a further agglomeration of ebony-layered buildings; in smoke-wrapped cuttings and tunnels.

A mournful place, London; characterized by memorials to the fallen. The awareness of some recent, appalling event began to loom on the periphery of my understanding, adumbrated by lugubrious effigies in stone and bronze – the iron soldier reading his iron letter at Paddington Station; the immobile greatcoated sentries at Hyde Park Corner standing guard over a corpse, a basinlike helmet laid on its breast; the inscribed plaques, whole walls incised with unending columns of names and initials; and everywhere those dates, 1914 and 1918.

I liked, however, the standard showplaces to which I was taken – Hampton Court, the Tower of London, and St Bartholomew's Church in Smithfield. But there was nothing to beat Madame Tussaud's Waxworks. I remember seeing the coach Napoleon used at Waterloo (this was before the fire which destroyed it). The Chamber of Horrors was my favourite. In those days it really was a chamber of horrors, no mere boring collection of wax statuary dressed up in the clobber of executed criminals. There was a severed head – done in wax of course – with an eyeball half torn out, dangling realistically from the bloody socket by a ligament. On one wall hung an instructive series of photographs of a Chinese execution, showing a kneeling prisoner in the act of being beheaded with a scimitar. I was much interested in the fountain of blood – a jet of six feet – spurting from the neck arteries at the moment of decapitation. There were other gruesomenesses, mostly to do with medieval torture, on exhibition. But when I last visited Madame Tussaud's a few years after the end of Hitler's war, all these things had been removed. None of the horrors I saw as a child gave me nightmares; I wondered why they were later considered too shocking for public exhibition, especially after the more horrible actrocities – genocide, Belsen, the gas-chambers of Auschwitz, Coventry, Dresden, Hiroshima – of the war we had just endured. Too near the bone perhaps?

Meanwhile I was going through my own small purgatory. That winter I ran the gauntlet of the ear-nose-and-throat men. My parents were ready to grasp at any straw that offered a chance of restoring my hearing. Most of these straws made themselves available for grasping, at a price, in Harley Street. Unfortunately my father had then plenty of money to dissipate on the consulting-rooms of that long canyon of false hope. Hope (though not mine) led me to doors behind which eminent men, specialists in their profession, rang tuning forks for me to listen to (no go); went to work with squirts and syringes; laid me on operating-couches and clubbed me over the vertebrae; pumped soapy water up my rectum; or strapped electrical pads to the backs of my ears. This last caper I found painless but boring, till one day the pads slipped and gave me a slight shock. I took good care to make out I had been all but electrocuted and so got off further treatment. What hope these carryings-on had of achieving anything I have no clue; but then I was not the one who listened to the sales-talk of the specialists. This ordeal was a testament of my parents' love and despair.

For me the experience was mildly traumatic. To this day I cannot walk in Harley Street without a depression of spirit. And I find it hard to hide exasperation when kind strangers come up with news of some revolutionary operation guaranteed to bring its victim once again within range of birdsong, etc. Such well-meaners are not to know that I would as soon put my head in a gas-oven as lay it down on an operating-table for some fancy surgeon to make bad worse. But to be fair, I was later to owe my life to Harley Street. In 1941 a doctor X-rayed my old mastoid operation and told me I would be dead in a twelvemonth unless I gave him a free hand with the scalpel. I had the good luck to have a friend who was a medical student at Guy's Hospital, who advised me to consult a certain Harley Street specialist. This man told me that another operation on my ear would be my death-warrant. I had no difficulty in believing this because a few years before a deaf friend of mine with similar mastoid trouble had undergone much the same operation that the surgeon recommended. Three months later he was dead.

But to conclude my experiences with the healing profession. My parents' search for a cure did not end till about 1930, when I was taken to a Johannesburg faith-healer. This faith-healer was a well-to-do old lady (judging from my memory of her house and garden). Her 'treatment' was innocuous; I had to sit in a chair for an hour or so at a stretch while she waved her hands over my head. At least it kept the flies off. Many years later this lady became the subject, or rather the heroine, of a book that set out to prove the existence of life after death. According to this work she was a highly successful spirit medium, a kind of telephone-exchange with limbo. As a healer her cures were said to be numberless.

By now I had been deaf for over a twelvemonth. Already my speech was beginning to blur. Though I could 'hear' my own voice I could not hear enough to monitor the sounds I produced. I was becoming unintelligible to strangers. My mother realized that something would have to be done or I must lapse into incoherence. She began to look round for a specialized teacher who could take me in hand.

At this point she had the good fortune to hear of a Miss Neville, a qualified teacher of the deaf who took private pupils.

When I knew her Miss Neville was silver-haired, straight-backed as an Edwardian duchess and as formidable. When she died some years ago I discovered from the obituary notice in the *Teacher of the Deaf* just how highly she was regarded in her profession and by everybody who had had the luck to be taught by her. I am forever in debt to this exceptional woman. Quite apart from rescuing me from inarticulateness she laid the foundations of my education. Until I went to her I had the barest smattering of the three R's. I could read, but barely form letters; as for arithmetic, I was as beasts that perish.

Miss Neville taught at a ground-floor flat, which was most probably also her private residence, in the pillared arcades of Regent's Park Crescent. At that time there was only one other pupil, a girl called Vanessa, slightly older than myself. None the less Miss Neville employed an assistant teacher, Miss Holland. Ruth Holland was of course a much younger woman than Miss Neville; hawk-nosed, with raven hair. She also was a first-rate teacher of the deaf.

We were taught orally. To begin with Miss Neville took my speech in hand, subjecting it to a daily drill. Next she completely reformed my handwriting. Under her I acquired a beautiful round cursive of which I now possess the seedy remains: laziness, the typewriter, and the system of punishment favoured by the schools I was afterwards to attend – the writing out of lines by the hundred – sapped it long ago. I even achieved a grasp of simple arithmetic, advancing as far as long division. Later in life I was to be instructed in more abstruse mathematical techniques, such as sums involving the highest common factor and lowest common multiple, though my understanding of these has now deserted me. But I can still do long division, and often as not get it right.

This is my first lesson with Miss Neville. I am alone with her in the room, slightly awed but ready to take advantage.

'Stand up,' says Miss Neville.

I stand up. This was good psychology. She began with an order, which I obeyed without thinking, and in so doing set the pattern of our future roles: Miss Neville's to tell me what to do, mine to do it.

'Say E.'

'E.'

'Say A.'

'A.'

'Now say E, A.'

'E, A.'

'Say S.'

'S.'

'Now say them all together – E, A, S.'

'E, A, S.'

'Very good. Repeat, EAS.'

'EAS.'

'Say it faster. EAS, EAS.'

'EAS, EAS, EAS, yes!'

I find myself saying 'yes' unawares.

'There you are, John. You can say "yes" perfectly.'

How simple, yet effective. With this technique, and a daily speech drill in which I had to repeat endlessly a litany of un-related monosyllables in order to exercise the pronunciation of different vowels and consonants, Miss Neville unlocked my tongue. It really felt like that.

Years later, reading the Penguin translation of Bede's *History of the English Church and People*, I was startled to come upon the following account of the 'miraculous' cure of a dumb youth by St John of Beverley:

When one week of Lent was past, on the following Sunday John told the poor fellow to come to him, and ordered him to put out his tongue and show it him; then he took him by the chin, and making the sign of the holy cross upon his tongue, told him to retract it and speak. 'Pronounce some word,' he said: 'say gae,' which is the English word of agreement and assent, i.e. 'Yes'. The young man's tongue was loose and at once he did what he was told. The bishop then proceeded to the names of letters: 'Say A,' he said. And he said 'A'. 'Now say B,' he said, which the youth did. And when he had repeated each of the letters after the bishop, the latter added syllables and words for him to repeat after him. When he had said all of them, he told him to repeat longer sentences, and he did so.

Making allowance for Bede's insistence on the miraculous, and for his probably having heard some more or less garbled account from someone who did not understand what the bishop was doing, it seems clear that St John taught his dumb youth to speak by means of a speech-drill and techniques basically the same as those Miss Neville had used upon me.

Sometimes I took lessons with Vanessa. She was the first deaf child I had met. We got on well enough together but neither found the other very interesting. She was fair-haired, rather pretty, and had a slightly stony expression. Like all Miss Neville's pupils she wrote a beautiful hand; she was much better than me at arithmetic. But even to an eight-year-old like myself her general knowledge seemed strangely limited. I remember a geography lesson we were doing together, when Miss Neville asked,

'Who is the king of England?'

Vanessa didn't know; troubled, she tried to read sideways the geography book, which lay open at the chapter about Great Britain that we had prepared.

'King – king,' began Vanessa.

'Go on,' commanded Miss Neville.

'I know,' I said.

'Be quiet.'

'United Kingdom,' said Vanessa.

I laughed.

'You are very silly,' said Miss Neville. 'How can a king be called "United Kingdom"?'

'King United Kingdom,' tried poor Vanessa, scarlet.

'Tell her if you know, John.'

'King George the Fifth,' I said proudly.

'It's not fair! It wasn't in the book!'

Vanessa was quite right of course; the chapter on the geography of Great Britain did not concern itself with its political set-up. She was far from stupid; but having been born deaf her slowly and painfully acquired vocabulary was still too small to allow her to read for amusement or pleasure. As a consequence there were almost no means by which she could pick up the fund of miscellaneous and temporarily useless information other children unconsciously acquire from conversation or random reading. Almost everything she knew she had been taught or made to learn. And this is a fundamental difference between hearing and deaf-born children – or was, in that pre-electronic era.

About this time I began writing my first verses; because I found I liked reading poetry, I began to want to make some of my own. Until I came to England the only verse I read had been nursery rhymes, A. A. Milne, and the kind of thing that used to get printed in children's annuals. In London I had come upon the poetry with which Kipling peppered his *Just-so Stories*, and the High Edwardian selection of 'Great Poems' in Arthur Mee's *Children's Encyclopedia*. It may be that if I had not become deaf I would not have troubled my head with the stuff. What I liked about poetry was what I called 'the tune' – the element of music I could express from metrically ordered language, rhythm and rhyme. There may have been a family inclination for music that I inherited. One of our Settler forebears is said to have been a musician; my father and both his sisters had even been sent to Dresden for a full-scale musical education. For myself I had been fond of music before I became deaf – the violin was my favourite instrument – yet I cannot recall feeling any particular sense of deprivation when I could no longer hear it. Perhaps I was too young to mind; perhaps I found a substitute in poetry.

In the spring or early summer of 1929 my mother and I returned to South Africa, sailing in the RMS *Themistocles*, the same boat that had brought us out the year before.* I was delighted to

*Long afterwards, talking with the poet Roy Campbell, I found that the ship in which he embarked for England in 1928 after the collapse of *Voorslag* (the 'little review' he edited with William Plomer and Laurens Van der Post) had been the *Themistocles*. If so we must have been shipmates.

be leaving England. Once we were out of the Bay of Biscay I used to stride up and down the windy boat-deck in the early mornings declaiming over and over again poems from the *Children's Encyclopedia* that I now found I knew by heart. One particular poem which I was never tired of chanting does credit, I think, to my taste: it was Cowper's *Loss of the Royal George*. I do not know how the other passengers felt about it.

My formal education had been given a first-rate start by Miss Neville; this was continued by her assistant, Miss Holland, who came out to South Africa to be my governess.

In the interim I went to a very small deaf school at Johannesburg. Perhaps it was not a school at all. I remember only a personable young woman, very amiable, who taught deaf children somewhere in the town: or perhaps she did not teach them but kept them occupied. As I was with her for so short a time – not more than two or three weeks I believe – I recall little except that we were taught almost nothing besides the making of raffiawork artefacts.

Apart from whatever natural inability I am saddled with, since then I have had an aversion to doing anything with my hands. To this day I cannot draw, or tie up a parcel properly if it comes to that. I remain far from proud of this manual impotence. But for a long time, dating from my attendance at this school, if it was a school, I refused on principle to learn or was deliberately bad at manipulative skills like carpentry, painting, and so on. Schools of this type, where the teacher was usually untrained – they probably do not exist nowadays – took the line of least resistance and while teaching their deaf pupils a little speech and lip-reading, concentrated on instruction in handicrafts. This seemed to me, even then, to be equating deafness with stupidity; and I resented it. So much so that I took cleverness with the hands to be a badge of deafness, and I would not wear that badge. Instead of being taught to use my head, because I was deaf I was being fobbed off with raffiawork. This may have been a crude and unfair reaction but it lasted.

It also led me, unreasonably, to resist my parents' forethought in attempting to turn me into a gamesman. They were afraid that deafness might prove a social handicap when I grew up. Social life as understood by the white bourgeoisie of South Africa centred on the playing of games. Even in those days half the suburban houses of Johannesburg had their own tennis-courts. As for Sunday golf, it was and probably still is a sacred ritual. If, my parents reasoned, I became a good games-player I would possess a social asset which must more than offset the social debit of deafness. It was a perfectly sound idea, thwarted only by their son's intractable dislike of golf and the persistent frivolity with which he approached the game of tennis. The trouble was that he tended to put golf and tennis in the same class as raffiawork – an occupation for dolts. It is with this sort of ingratitude children reward their parents.

When some months later Miss Holland arrived in Johannesburg, she built firmly on the foundations of my education as laid down by Miss Neville. For a year or so I believe I was given a far better and more thorough education than I could possible have obtained at a school, even if I had been able to hear. As Miss Holland's sole pupil I had all her attention. Apart from being a trained teacher of the deaf she was an excellent all-round instructress. I believe that by the time she had finished with me I was in advance of most children of my age. This served me well when she had to leave us, for there were to be three years in which my education was sporadic and sketchy.

Four

All words are modified undulations of air,
made significant to the mind,
by social compact, or consent.

FRANCIS GREEN *Vox Oculis Subjecta*

1929, the year of the Wall Street crash, saw the end of the stock-broking firm of O. D. Wright & Son. Both my father and grandfather were ruined. Our house at Mountain View was sold up, with practically every stick of furniture. We moved to a rented cottage consisting of two rondavels (a rondavel is a small circular one-room building with a thatched roof) linked by an open stoep; to this a kitchen and bathroom had been tacked on. One of the rondavels served as a bedroom for my parents. The other became the sitting-room. The open stoep, which was roofed, had a bed put in it where I slept winter and summer. A tiny gas-stove furnished the kitchen; hot water for the bath was supplied by a homicidal wood-fired geyser. A far cry from the mansion where we had lived at Mountain View, yet we found it more of a home.

When we moved to the Rondavels (as the cottage was called) our fortunes were at rockbottom. Every morning my father set off on foot to catch the tram to the city centre, to return depressed and grim in the evening. Like everyone else he was looking for a job. My mother did much to make ends meet by turning her hospital training to account and assisting a local doctor as a midwife. Those were the first days of the great depression. Things cannot have been nearly as bad in South Africa as elsewhere, but they were bad. Just how bad was brought home to me one day when I saw a gang of labourers by the roadside digging a ditch for laying drainpipes. They were white men.*

* So what? This is a book about deafness, but as it is in part autobiography I have to digress. Like all Caucasoid South African children I had been unconsciously and therefore thoroughly conditioned to the caste system of the society to which I was born. Thus the spectacle of white men reduced to doing 'kaffir s work was traumatic – a reversal of the order of things as

By 1931 things began to pick up, at least for my father, who after trying for a variety of jobs obtained what they now call an executive post in the Legal & General, then beginning to operate in South Africa. After the winding-up of the family stock-broking firm he had not, of course, been able to continue employing Miss Holland as my full-time governess. I ran more or less wild, and spent most of my time with my friend Billy, who lived next door to our old home in Mountain View. We explored abandoned mine-shafts in the kopje; we experimented with the manufacture of gunpowder. We nearly broke our necks in the one and almost blew ourselves up with the other.

But if I was not getting much in the way of regular education I was confirmed in the habit of reading. My aunt Mat used to

hitherto understood. As a result, for the first time I began to suspect that white men and black belonged not only to the same creation but to the same species. This seems naïve, to say no worse: but reporting my attitude at the age of nine may throw light on though not excuse the intractability of South African and Rhodesian colour prejudice. The colour feeling of white South Africans is almost irremediable because irrational, built-in at birth and thereafter fostered as it were by the air they breathe. Black men are not seen as human beings but a sort of superior animal – the most highly developed of the local fauna. White South Africans may be attached to individual Africans, even love them dearly, but with few exceptions that love is of the same kind as love for a dog or horse. For, setting aside apartheid laws, the average white South African would no more dream of sitting down to table or eating from the same set of dishes and cutlery as his black friend, than he would of dining from 'the dog's plate'. A physical repulsion, the more terrible and commanding because involuntary and rooted elsewhere than in reason, forbids. It was by deliberate effort that I had to rid myself, long after I had left Africa, of this appalling insensitivity to which I had all my childhood been conditioned: an insensitivity to the humanity of one's fellow-creatures, to which is coupled an absurd, though equally appalling, sensitivity to the pigment of their skins. De Tocqueville in his monograph on the French Revolution noted that aristocratic ladies, though brought up to the standards of strictest modesty, thought nothing of undressing and stripping stark naked in front of their footmen: simply because it did not occur to them that a servant counted as a man. Much the same is true of the white South African's attitude to black Africans (how many symptoms that de Tocqueville noted as prognostications of the Revolution are observable in South Africa today). For instance, when I was sixteen it suddenly occurred to me to wonder why I did not find the spectacle of naked black women erotic (in the bushveld they are often to be seen bathing or washing by the side of a river). The answer was in de Tocqueville: like any pre-Revolutionary aristocrat I had been conditioned not to think of 'inferiors' as human.

send me from England books for Christmas and birthdays. These were substantial fare, at least by twentieth-century standards, for a child of my age, but reflected my aunt's solid Victorian-Scottish upbringing. They included *Pickwick Papers*, *Rob Roy*, *Guy Mannering*, *Moby Dick*, George Borrow's *Lavengro*, and the like; and must have done wonders for my vocabulary. All the same, my parents began to worry about my schooling.

The Rondavels stood at the foot of the same range of kopjes as our former home. Directly above the cottage, on the skyline of the hill, a huge and rococo edifice dominated the landscape. This was 'Tracy's Folly', built by a Rand millionaire of that name in the early 1900s. This gigantic mansion – almost a palace – looked north over the veld towards Pretoria and the Magaliesberg. It was a landmark for miles around. The architecture could be called Dutch Colonial, sort of; but on a colossal scale, as if the basic design of one of the gabled Dutch farmhouses at the Cape had been blown up to five or six times life-size. No less than eight enormous whitewashed gables faced the Magaliesberg. These curlicued fantasies were linked by a stone-balustraded stoep overhanging an almost sheer drop, for the house had been built on what was more or less a cliff. Its interior was an exercise in the grandiose and absurd: for example, the great panelled dining-hall containing a pair of carved, crushingly ornate, twisting pillars of Burmese teak lit by huge stained-glass windows illustrated with the arms of Tracy. This South African Gatsby never lived there, but died or went bankrupt, or both, soon after the place had been completed. Then it had been taken over by a private preparatory school called P.T.S. (the initials stood for Park Town School, Park Town being the suburb where it had originally been situated). It was a boarding-school – the pupils came from all parts of South Africa and Rhodesia – but accepted day-boys who had their homes in Johannesburg. It was this conveniently handy establishment that my parents decided I should attend.

In those days it was usual for bourgeois South Africans to send their sons to England at the age of thirteen or fourteen to complete their education at one of the public schools, and perhaps go on to Oxford or Cambridge. P.T.S. specialized in preparing its pupils for this programme. Thus it was very English indeed and run as nearly as possible on public-school lines: the masters were all English-educated, with or without university degrees. Its headmaster, R. G. L. Austin, was the apotheosis of a late Victorian English gentleman, or perhaps Edwardian would be nearer the mark. He wore an expression of dignified sadness above a cropped and greying moustache; was dressed invariably in an impeccably cut pepper-and-salt tweed suit. Above his study mantelpiece hung an overpowering signed photograph of W. G. Grace, bearded like the pard. The bookshelves (from which we were encouraged to borrow) were stacked with manly, cold-bath-in-the-morning, boys' books by Henty, Ballantyne, W. H. G. Kingston, and Talbot Baines Reed; humour being represented by Jerome K. Jerome and the exotic by Jules Verne, the animal stories of Ernest Thompson Seton and Charles G. D. Roberts. The school and its headmaster were so English they seemed a parody.*

It was an imaginative and generous decision on the part of the headmaster of P.T.S. when he agreed to allow me to become a pupil. The problems of having a deaf boy in a class of hearing pupils must have seemed formidable. On one hand he could not be allowed to hold up the rest of the class; on the other he could not be disregarded and more or less left to his own devices. In the end they must have decided to play it by ear, and see what happened.

The school ran to between sixty and a hundred pupils, most of them boarders. I was placed in the fourth form, a class of a dozen or so eleven-year-olds. I could follow blackboard work, and was all right in anything that involved the reading of texts or schoolbooks. The masters took trouble to write down necessary explanations for me – to give a modicum of individual tuition in fact – but I do not think they allotted me an unfair proportion of their time. However it was in subjects like Latin, French, and mathematics, where oral guidance and explanation is a great help, that I did worst; I failed to pick up anything worth a rap.

*The Englishness of this school tempts me to another digression. If the operation of colour-feeling cut off the average white South African from any contact, other than on a master–servant basis, with the black and coloured population, the division of white schools into English-speaking and Afrikaans-speaking establishments segregated the two white races almost as effectively – at least during childhood and adolescence. I do not think I met more than a dozen or so Afrikaner South Africans in the two preparatory schools I attended at Johannesburg. When I look back at my childhood in South Africa I am struck by the thoroughgoing way in which the divisions among its peoples were propagated and entrenched by the separate education of their children.

But thanks to Miss Neville and Miss Holland I had a solid grounding in history, geography, scripture, English, and so on, and was well able to keep up with the rest of the class where these were concerned.

Among the boys I was for a while a curiosity, interesting because of my deafness; then the novelty wore off and I found my friends and enemies like anybody else. Most of my time at P.T.S. I thoroughly enjoyed, though perhaps I might not have liked it so much had I been a boarder instead of a day-boy. The world of school had its problems which I could forget in the world of home; and vice versa. Deafness did not earn me any particularly special treatment, among the boys at least; though some of the staff may have refrained from clouting my head when my head needed clouting. So far as I can judge and remember, I was neither popular nor unpopular. At games I was useless; but the school, rather surprisingly, had no real games fetish and it was not held against me.*

My only problem, or at least the one that put all others out of my head, was that of the rest of the eleven-year-olds in my class. This was the bullying we had to undergo from some of the seniors. Not that it was anything on the scale of *Tom Brown's Schooldays* or *Stalky & Co.* There were, however, two notorious thugs. The worser, whom I will call Salt, was a dedicated artist in the various limb-wrenchings, constrictions, holds, and other sleights for the infliction of agony without leaving a mark. A favourite diversion of his was to make one of us turn a half-somersault so that the trunk balanced on the nape of the neck; whereupon Salt would seat himself smartly on the boy's upturned buttocks, throwing his entire weight on the spine of his victim, and thereby produce an excruciating spasm along the vertebrae. Nobody got a neck or a back broken, which seems a miracle. The other bully was a hanger-on of Salt's called Filey; not in himself vicious, just a loutish disciple. This pair were about fourteen years old; their victims, ten or eleven.

Their reign came to a sudden end. One of those long Saturday

---

*One of my friends, a redhaired bullet-headed freckle-faced type, became the best cricketer the school ever produced – N. B. F. Mann, who played for South Africa. A slow but mortally accurate bowler, he was the best of his class I ever saw – but that was at Lord's, a decade and a half later. At school he was regarded as a batsman. He died of cancer before he was thirty.

half-holiday afternoons when there were no organized games, a group of us smaller boys began talking about all we had suffered at the hands of Salt and Filey. Then something came over us – a panic visitation of rage. For the first and I hope last time I had the experience of being incorporated into the body of a mob – the self actually subsumed into the being of something other and monstrous. There were a dozen or more of us. We were Circefied: turned into an animal. Not animals, but a single animal made up of all. As by some communal decision a flock of starlings will suddenly take to the air in a body, as suddenly we began to pick up anything that would serve for a weapon: rulers, sticks, cricket-stumps, bats, a board wrenched from a broken box. Armed with these we went in search of Salt. We had no interest in Filey.

Salt we found in the nets at batting practice. He was no chickenheart (the superstition that bullies are cowards doesn't bear looking at). Small as we were, we must have been intimidating – a score of us brandishing sticks and staves (for we had picked up recruits on the way), obviously out for blood. But Salt kept his head. He said nothing, but leant on his bat and looked at us one by one. He smiled a little. And we halted: that cold eye like a snake's quelled us. Having faltered, we were beaten. One by one we turned around and began to retreat the way we had come. We straggled back along the winding gravel drive to the schoolhouse, when as his bad luck would have it Salt's hanger-on, Filey, who was the less formidable of the two, came round the corner on his way to the nets. We were totally unexpected; Filey had no warning; and to the fury in possession of us had been added fury at our ignominy in the face of Salt. There and then, without a word, we fell on Filey; I saw him disappear under a cloud of flailing sticks and bats. How he escaped being killed I cannot explain.

I don't really remember what happened after we ran into Filey. Perhaps a master came by and rescued him before we could do much damage. He was taken to the sanatorium, that I know; and reappeared a day or two later, chastened and sticking-plastered. The curious thing about this incident is that it seemed to have no repercussions. The staff may have known or guessed what had been going on, and taken the line that Filey had got what was coming to him. Though it was not Filey, but Salt, whom we were after.

None of us ever discussed or even referred to what had happened. We returned to our individual selves ashamed and purged, and never spoke about it. There was, by the by, no more bullying. Salt and Filey left school at the end of that term, and they had no successors.

I had begun writing poetry about a year after I became deaf, when I was eight. At twelve, I was still writing verse. None of my friends at school or elsewhere could have been called bookish; I wrote without encouragement or discouragement. The miscellany of books at home included Kipling's *Barrack-Room Ballads*, a lot of R. W. Service, the inevitable *Rubaiyat of Omar Khayyám*, the poems of Browning and W. E. Henley. There was also a copy of *Hamlet*, which I couldn't understand a word of. One of the school textbooks was Palgrave's *Golden Treasury, with Additional Poems*. This I read over and over again, not only during the English lesson but all the others, whenever I could get away with it. My enthusiasms in poetry were conventional – Shelley's *Skylark*, the glories of our blood and state, a little Wordsworth, Tennyson's *Revenge* and Browning's *Hervé Riel* (a much better poem by the way). Another, perhaps unlikely, source of poetry I found in *Hymns Ancient and Modern*, which I got to know well by dint of reading the hymnal as a time-killer during morning prayers. I would have read more had the books been available. The headmaster's library – or at least that part of it open to the scrutiny of his pupils – I have already described. There was no public library where I could browse. (The Johannesburg Public Library stood in the city centre, where I was not allowed to go unaccompanied for fear of the traffic.) With two or three exceptions, few of our neighbours and friends possessed more than a couple of dozen books, and these were mostly an unvarying miscellany of interchangeable titles. The houses of the majority of Johannesbourgeois in the thirties seem to have been nearly as bookless as the English working-class homes described in Richard Hoggart's *The Uses of Literacy*.

If anybody is responsible for my deciding, later, that my vocation was poetry, it must be one of the masters at P.T.S., though he might be surprised to hear it. This was the English and history master, J. W. O. Fuller. He was an enthusiast who communicated enthusiasm. Under him, each term we read a play of Shakespeare's, which he made come alive by getting us to act the scenes, usually out of doors on the lawn beside the swimming-pool. If he did not distil much of the sort of information acceptable to the setters of examination-papers, he at least made an association between literature and enjoyment. Mr Fuller was the first person I ever met for whom books and ideas were a passion. He never talked down to me. As he walked along he would jot his remarks on bits of paper and backs of envelopes (he being one of the many people I could never learn to lipread) on subjects ranging from H. G. Wells to the partition of Ireland. A dangerous man, in love with the idea of writing, over which he threw a cloak of glamour. He told me not to do as he had done.

'Shaw said, "Those who can't, teach." Remember the Witch: "I'll do and I'll do and I'll do".'

He gave me the run of his collection of books – not more than a shelf-ful or two, all that he had been able to bring out with him from England, but to me new and strange. This 'library' was quite free of the usual best-sellers, half-hearted, unopened 'classics', golf manuals, gardening encyclopedias and volumes whose titles began *With Rod and Gun*, or *In Darkest*, and other hardy perennials of Johannesburg drawing-rooms. Some of these books he not only lent but gave me – those I still have juxtapose oddly: Naomi Mitchison's *The Conquered*, the complete works of Saki, and Oswald Spengler's *Decline of the West*.

When he talked of books he talked of their writers, most of whose names I had never heard – for that reason they seemed all the more glamorous. Out of school I pestered him with questions, hoping to start one of his long rambling paper disquisitions which might begin with Manchuria and end with Aldous Huxley. I must have been a nuisance; on at least one occasion, as I long afterwards realized, an embarrassment. What, I wanted to know, did Oscar Wilde go to jail for? Mr Fuller evaded the question; naturally I kept returning to it. At this time – it was before the days of paperback sex – I had no notion, not even a birds and bees one, of the facts of life. Finally he told me that if I wanted to know I would have to ask the headmaster. Mystified and more curious than ever, I waylaid that kindly old man one afternoon as he strolled in the garden.

'Please sir, what did Oscar Wilde go to jail for?'

Mr Austin beckoned me to follow him. To the schoolhouse he led me, and thence into his study. Settling himself behind his desk he took his gold spectacles out of their case and balanced them carefully upon his nose; unscrewed his fountain-pen and wrote on a piece of paper, which he handed me in silence. It bore one word: 'Immorality'.

Five

As if Man had another mouth
or fountain of discourse in his Hand.
DR JOHN BULWER, *Chirologia*

AT the age of thirteen I left South Africa; as it turned out, for good.

The problem that faced my parents from the moment I lost my hearing had been my education. Obviously I could not go to an ordinary school. They had been lucky in finding as brilliant a teacher of the deaf as Miss Neville, and through her, so able a governess as Miss Holland. The preparatory school at Johannesburg represented an agreeable and in some ways valuable interlude but was no more than a temporary solution. Where was I to go from there? This was a hard question to answer if, as my parents had always intended, I was to go to a university. My deafness appeared to have knocked that dream on the head.

Private tuition might have been the answer. But it would have meant isolation from contemporaries. In any case my parents could not have afforded it.

There were schools for the deaf in South Africa but none attempted much more than elementary education for deaf children. In fact there was only one school for the deaf in the British Commonwealth able to provide an education up to university level for its pupils. This English school, unique then and for many years afterwards, had been founded by a nineteenth-century pioneer of deaf education, the Rev. Thomas Arnold. He was no relation of that other great headmaster, his namesake, but in his own field had been hardly less influential, and hardly less renowned. Arnold's great triumph had been the education of Abraham Farrar,* the first pupil from a deaf school ever to enter a

* Abraham Farrar (1861–1944) was born at Leeds, and entered London University in 1881, where he qualified as an architect and surveyor, though he never practised. Farrar helped Arnold to write the monumental sccond edition of his *Education of Deaf Mutes: A Manual for Teachers* (1888)

university and take a degree. Farrar was still alive while my parents were debating what to do about educating me. This may suggest how new a phenomenon the higher education of the deaf then was, and for that matter still is.

Arnold's establishment, which he described as a 'middle-class school for the deaf and dumb', had been launched in 1868 at Northampton. It was a private school, whose headmaster, Frederick Ince-Jones, the third in succession to the founder, had been its principal for a quarter of a century. Under this remarkable man the school had flourished along the lines laid down by Arnold, and had gained an academic record second to none in the deaf world. It is a record that must look pathetic by ordinary standards, but epoch-making in the sphere of deaf education. When the school closed down for ever in 1944 its achievement included, besides scores of successes in lesser public examinations, thirteen pupils who had matriculated and six who had taken university degrees.

The school at Northampton offered my best hope of getting into a university. So, at a personal and financial sacrifice which I was then far from understanding or appreciating, my parents made up their minds to send me there. Among other things it entailed for them another long separation. While my father remained in Johannesburg my mother would have to take me to Northampton, since they did not think I could travel the six thousand miles to England alone.

In 1934 people followed Jim Mollison's flights across the Atlantic with bated breath. Nowadays one flies to England from Johannesburg in a few hours, but in the thirties the only route was by sea. Our voyage to England, when I look back on it, seems a period piece. I might as well be recalling hansom-cabs and horse-buses. But it was a splendid voyage, with vicissitudes.

We embarked a few days after Christmas at Lourenço Marques in Portuguese East Africa, travelling for cheapness' sake in a German boat, the *Adolph Woermann*. She was to follow the East Coast route via the Red Sea, Suez, and the Mediterranean. She flew

---

and after Arnold's death was responsible for the revision and rewriting of this standard work, the latest edition of which appeared in 1954. Farrar contributed much valuable research on the history of the education of the deaf in the course of a long life.

the Nazi flag: it was the year that Hitler came into power. Before we embarked my father remarked:

'Be careful. The Germans have a man called Hitler. I don't know anything about him but the Germans think he's God. If you try to be funny you'll get into trouble.'

My father accompanied us to the ship. He made straight for the smoking-room, hoping for a glass of Munich beer. Alas for him the bar was closed in port. He said good-bye at once – he could not bear farewells; this was to be a long parting. From the boat deck I watched him hasten his dot-and-carry limp, not once looking back, across the dustbrown quay to the harbour gates.

My mother and I travelled third-class, sharing a steel-partitioned compartment rather bigger than a golf-club locker. Our fellow-voyagers were mostly middle-aged Germans though a few English and South Africans sprinkled the passenger-list. One feature of life aboard the *Adolph Woermann* was the superfluity and weirdness of meals – passengers were summoned to a groaning table every three hours – another, the sullen resentfulness of her crew. The atmosphere of the ship was rebarbative. Glass cases in which tourist brochures would normally have been displayed were bleak with Teutonic propaganda. The title of each book and pamphlet revolved about the word Versailles, while skulls, bayonets, barbed wire and bloodstained daggers enlivened the dustcovers. You could see that the Germans were not pleased at having lost the war. Even to me it was obvious that the next one could not be far off.

But as it turned out the *Adolph Woermann* carried us less than half-way to England. At Zanzibar I went down with malaria. Almost simultaneously my mother contrived to have an accident: climbing out of her bunk one night she pitched to the floor and broke her arm. Next morning the pair of us were dumped on the quay at Mombasa – my mother in pink dressing-gown with her arm in a sling, myself in pyjamas and sun-helmet. A rickshaw trundled us to hospital while the German boat steamed off.*

At Mombasa we were stranded a fortnight or more in a hospital that stood hard by an old Portuguese fort overlooking the channel. We might have been in awkward case had not a Mr and Mrs White, hearing by chance of our predicament, made our

* A few years later I was to read in *The Times* of the sinking of the *Adolph Woermann*; after a chase by a British warship, she scuttled herself somewhere in the middle of the South Atlantic.

troubles their own. We had not even the claim of a common acquaintance; nevertheless they visited us at hospital, showered books and flowers and fruit-cake, and as soon as we were convalescent took us for drives round the island. Of Mombasa all I remember is the dhows with scimitar sails, the camels, mangoes, baobab trees, and the habit some native women had of slinging their great pendulous breasts over their shoulders for ease when walking. And, of course, the disinterested and indefatigable generosity of our good Samaritans, who even arranged the transfer of our passage to the next boat sailing for Europe.

She was the *Llanstephan Castle*, a slow but comfortable old tub – the same ship that had taken my parents out to South Africa when they married. In contrast to the millimetre-pinching design of the German boat she was distinguished, even in her tourist quarters, by Edwardian commodiousness and elegance – a sort of sunset-of-empire afterglow. There was a sort of sunset-of-empire afterglow about the passengers too: notably Colonel Copeman.

To this peppery old vexillary I represented suffering and penance. His passion was backgammon, which game (having despaired of finding any other opponent) the Colonel taught me on his own private leather-bound gold-tooled backgammon board. Thereafter I was condemned to thrice-daily sessions in the tourist smoking-room, where we rattled dice and positioned our men, where six times an hour the Colonel called on God to witness the nadir of human imbecility: paroxysmic detonations brought about by the exasperation of a master pitted against a novice. Tough and lean as a piece of old biltong, the Colonel terrorized the tourist class. A devastating individualist, he could and would rout the ship's jolly-boy – the deck-games organizer – or sober up the ship's drunk with a basilisk stare from the backgammon board. To which he chained me night and day, except for periods of release while he did his exercises. The Colonel was improving his eyesight by the Bates method.

This system involved what he called 'palming' – the Colonel sitting with head bent, nursing his eyeballs in the heels of his hands for as much as an hour at a stretch. Another article of the treatment would bring him up to the boat deck to relax with rigid concentration on a deck chair, eyes shut tight in order to allow the beneficent rays of the sun to do their stuff on the closed lids. This would be followed by a definitely alarming exercise wherein he sat bolt upright as if in cataleptic trance, motionless except for a clockwork swivelling of the eyeballs. But the Bates system worked. When the Colonel came aboard at Mombasa he could barely read the daily menu even when thrust against his nose. By the time we disembarked at Tilbury he was holding it at arm's length, sarcastically declaiming items for the benefit of the head steward:

'Canton pudding. Ha! Madeira pudding Monday, Boston pudding Tuesday, Valparaiso pudding Wednesday. As if we didn't know it's that damn spotted dick. Bloody fool!'

The *Llanstephan Castle* grunted her way up a wintry Red Sea, through the Canal, past the white cliffs of Crete and red volcanic blink of Stromboli. She gave us a February day at Genoa where we visited the fantastic cemetery at Staglieno; coasted along the Riviera, calling at Marseilles. Gibraltar, Tangier, Cape St Vincent; a wallow across the Bay of Biscay and there we were, at Tilbury and England.

So it was in dead of winter, on a tenebrous afternoon, I arrived at Northampton. It was my fourteenth birthday. Term was nearly half done; I had missed its first weeks because of our inadvertent stopover at Mombasa.

The taxi from the station had taken us through the centre of the town, past soon-to-be-familiar All Saints' with its statue of Charles II in Roman toga and peruke, a Victorian town hall and dun-coloured general hospital. The school turned out to be a solid nineteenth-century stuccoed brick mansion with a pillared portico standing in what, before the speculative deposits of the early thirties, had been an outer suburb of Northampton. The house hid behind tall hedges of thick yew and holly.

A maid in cap and apron, white face slashed with a purple harelip, answered the bell. My mother and I were shown into a cluttered, pleasantly chintzy, firelit sitting-room, where the principal and his wife awaited us. Yet I remember nothing of this first encounter with that extraordinary Welshman of the gold monocle, Augustan features, prescriptive will, implacable charm, obsessive patience and fiery choler. All impressions were blotted out by my introduction, half an hour later, to that other world to which I belonged but was yet to enter.

This new life began as soon as I had said good-bye to my mother. I was ushered along a dark cupboardy passage that led to the dining-room. It was late afternoon, or early evening. The senior boys were at supper, the one meal of the day not presided over by any member of the staff. This accident plunged me *in medias res* among my future companions, uninhibited by the presence of authority or of outsiders from the hearing world. Up till then I had had no contact to speak of with the deaf. This was my initiation to their freemasonry. I went in at the deep end.

A long table at the back of the dining-room seats perhaps a dozen boys. Is the verb right? Confusion stuns the eye, arms whirl like windmills in a hurricane, thunderous unbroken drumming assaults what's left of the ear. Heelthuds shake the floor while someone hammers on the table. Mouths frame words: vowels and consonants blown up like photographic enlargements, every syllable reinforced by the emphatic silent vocabulary of the body – look, expression, bearing, glance of eye; hands perform their pantomime. Absolute engrossing pandemonium. Nothing I was ever to come across in later life held a candle to this scene – not even the saloon bars and late-night caffs of Soho and Fitzrovia in the forties. Yet this is a normal supper (at other meals, under the eye of the staff, behaviour is circumscribed) such as I am to participate in every evening for the next five years, and never turn a hair.

I begin to sort out what's going on. The seemingly corybantic brandishing of hands and arms reduces itself to a convention, a code which as yet conveys nothing. It is in fact a kind of vernacular. The school has evolved its own peculiar language or argot, though not a verbal one.

Tableau: an argument is going on. Two boys try to impress their points of view on a third, who won't listen, but defends his opinion by keeping downturned eyes fixed upon his plate. Did he glance up he might read the words they were saying and be lost. The other two, one on each side, hammer their knuckles against either shoulder to make him look up. Realizing he won't, one of them grabs his head, wrenches it round till the eyes are level with his mouth. This idea is taken up by the other, who now seizes the head and jerks it back again to point at his own face. Owner of head bears the manhandling with perfect indifference and perfect determination not to be communicated with. He has screwed his eyes tight shut.

Around this contretemps the meal proceeds. At supper everyone is allowed to bring his own provender, which may be anything from sardines to cocoa, pickled onions, cake, cornflakes, tinned pineapple, jam, dates, God knows what. While apparently engaging every limb and feature in the service of communication, all simultaneously prepare and dispatch the food in front of them, offering one another fruit and cake and biscuits, slopping milk and sugar over bowls of cereal. It's like watching a three-ring circus.

This has taken time to describe, but in fact I am not given more than a moment to absorb the spectacle before being – well, not introduced, but sucked into the irresistible maelstrom of energy pulsating round the supper-table. Remarks are shot at and about me, eatables pressed hospitably into my hands.

To reproduce their talk by transcribing no more than the words actually used must misrepresent and distort its quality. Its life and subtlety (the observation and humour were often subtle) depended on expressive demeanour, face, and eye, on mimic gift: the pantomimic gesture subsuming a cartoonist's graphic ability to seize, magnify, and focus some essential point. The words constitute perhaps twenty per cent of the means of communication; their job seems mainly to specify or pinpoint what's being discussed. Gesture and expression then take over, to elaborate and qualify. A framework of spoken nouns is enough – mime does the work of a verb, a grimace offers the adjective. On the basis of one uttered vocable may be erected whole sentences and paragraphs.

But for the record I set down the words as spoken, running together in a single paragraph the contributions of half-a-dozen speakers, the remarks made to or at me, as they came:

'John Wright. From South Africa. Brown! Brown! Look, brown! Hot! Look! BRRROWN! (They were admiring my African suntan, which must have looked rather conspicuous in February.) Sun! Whew! Do you like girls? Shut up! I'm tired of you! I'm talking! Plymouth, me. Jimmy Boyce is South African. Jimmy! Jimmy! Shut up! Listen to me! I'm talking to John Wright. Jimmy Boyce is Johannesburg! Do you like England? Rain, rain, wet, cold, dark, sad, sad, no fruit. This is William. He is very poor. This is Julian Watson. He is Head Prefect. Jimmy has a girl friend. True! True! This is Henry Garnet. He is mad. Mad. Yes you are. MAD. Shut up! Wrong, wrong! Thought! You THOUGHT! Have you seen the king? I saw the king. This is Dermot. Clever. Brains, brains. Dermot has a letter from the king. Mad! Mad! Not the king. Buckingham Palace. I saw! I saw! Shut up! Be quiet! I'm tired of you! Do you like swimming? We swim in summer. Down there at Midsummer Meadow. Girls not allowed. Very sad! Very SA–A–A–D! Very MEL–ANCH–O–LY!'

The last speaker would have been Charles Oakley, a boy of doleful countenance, given to the collection of polysyllabic vocables and extraordinary epithets, most of which he picked up in the Shakespeare class. (I remember one day, when I had annoyed him, he turned upon me and remarked with lugubrious deliberation: 'Hag-seed!')

The deaf-and-dumb alphabet we never used; it was strictly against the rules of the school. Most of the pupils, like myself, had never even learnt it. All communications were supposed to be oral. Our own sign-argot was of course prohibited, like another habit we had of not using the voice when forming words (it makes for easier lipreading apart from the obvious advantage of cutting the risk of being overheard). But these rules could not be enforced without the presence of the staff. What I have been describing is not how we talked, but how we talked among ourselves when no hearing person was present. At such times our behaviour and conversation were quite different. We relaxed inhibitions, wore no masks. But the presence of the hearing naturally constrained our modes of communication. Besides, in front of hearing people we would try to appear 'normal'.

The Northampton school consisted of about a score of pupils representing all ages between seven and twenty-three. Some were only partially deaf, some like myself had had a few years of hearing before deafness overtook them. These two categories almost always had a larger vocabulary than those who had had the bad luck to be born profoundly deaf and had thus not begun to learn to speak or even understand language till they were three or four years old. Among us, therefore, existed differences of range and vocabulary when it came to spoken language. Some, not necessarily the youngest, could command no more than a couple of dozen words, mostly nouns; at the other extreme, several had a more or less average mastery of the language. Among ourselves we naturally tended to speak in a form that could be understood by the least articulate. The principle of the lowest common denominator operated here as elsewhere. Our peculiar argot of signs and gestures in fact derived from those of us whose verbal equipment was the smallest.

Idiosyncratic gestures that had originated with some barely articulate fellow-pupil (who might long ago have left school, but whose vocabulary of signs had survived his going) were propagated by use, as words are. Some bore little apparent relation to their meaning – for example, rubbing the breastbone with the tips of the fingers meant 'I didn't do it'. I give this example because I know its etymology, so to speak; it derived from a gesture used by Henry Garnet, who could utter perhaps three or four words. This wizened creature, whose deafness and feeble frame had been due to premature birth and to his mother's undernourishment in the First World War, was the most backward of the boys. Many people might have thought him mentally deficient, but they would have been wrong. The gesture was one of his habits. He would rub his chest in that way while trying to utter the word 'Good'. This meant, or stood for, 'I am a good boy'* – which was also his way of saying 'I didn't do it'. Now I come to think of it, much of our semeiology – if that be the proper term for sign language – emanated from Henry Garnet.

We also had nicknames, non-verbal nicknames; abbreviated mimes indicating a salient feature or idiosyncrasy – rather like the selective exaggeration of caricature. Because the headmaster wore an eyeglass his 'nickname' became a caliper movement of thumb and forefinger (originally it had been a proper round O made with finger and thumb and applied to the eye) – a shorthand reference to the famous monocle. Or a habit would do – the assistant master, Mr Mundin, had a trick of fingering his chin: which characteristic gesture, much stylized, became his appellation. Some were satiric; Jimmy Boyce would be indicated by a quick mime: index finger wipes dewdrop from the nose. A fist clenched at the back of the head, fingers exploding upwards, became my 'nickname'; this was supposed to imitate the way my unbrushed hair stuck out.

It was a tribal language. More than a quarter of a century after I had left Northampton and almost forgotten the life there, I was twice brought back to it – or rather had recreated for me the ambience of that time. On the first occasion I was sitting outside a café at Olhão, a small fishing port in Algarve. A few lads animatedly talking, using the electric gesticulations characteristic of the Olhãoenses, caught my attention. There was something familiar, something I could not quite put a finger on; I felt a

* Henry Garnet had a large *written* vocabulary, and would often write that sentence down; but the only word of it he could pronounce (or attempt to pronounce) was 'Good' – at least for his first year or so at school.

nostalgic Proustian emanation – and realized that the youths were deaf, that they were using the same kind of semaphore mime as ours at Northampton. I watched them for a long time without being able to find out what they were talking about. This didn't surprise me. They were using their own dumb-crambo argot which would be incomprehensible to anyone outside their own group, just as ours was. As will be seen, the fact that I could not speak Portuguese had nothing to do with my inability to follow what they were saying. For on the second occasion, about a year later, I was at Rome, having dinner in a little side street taberna off the Piazza Navona which had become my local. A party of about a dozen people came in and took a table next to mine. Again that sense of familiarity; in a moment or two I guessed that they were deaf. As soon as they had finished their meal I introduced myself as *'Inglese sordo.'** None of them spoke English, while I had two words of Italian, one of which was *sordo* and the other *scusa*. The party was a deaf-and-dumb club from the Piazza Gesù having its annual dinner. The president was a garage hand from Ostia; the others were tailors, carpenters, seamstresses. All this they told me with a few fluent movements. Our communications by-passed language. On one level I understood what they said better than a hearing Italian could have – and vice versa; we belonged after all to a country bounded by the same silent frontier. Towards the end of the evening we got considerably excited and the dinner took on the pattern of the school suppers at Northampton. At one stage the proprietor began to get alarmed; I don't blame him. He thought we were drunk. He was also much taken aback by the unexpected transmogrification of his quiet *scrittore inglese* into an apparently lunatic deaf-mute.

To return to my installation at Northampton. As soon as supper was over (it lasted twenty minutes) I was led to the schoolroom, which was contained in a block of brick outbuildings – probably a converted stables – separated from the house. It was a long, rectangular, green-painted room with a coal fire burning in a grate at the far end. Over its mantelpiece hung a framed, hand-painted Roll of Honour on which were inscribed the names of all the pupils who had passed public examinations. Most entries were for Oxford Junior Locals, a few for School Certificates, and three or four for university degrees – among them Abraham Farrar, the school's first pupil. There were about forty names on the list. In

* 'Deaf Englishman' – bad Italian but intelligible.

the middle of the room had been placed a yellow-brown photo-graph of the founder, the Rev. Thomas Arnold. His Victorian line-aments – a strong-nosed clean-shaven face set above a white bushy fluff that flourished below the jawline like a fur muffler – glared at a blackboard running the length of the opposite wall. Fifteen or sixteen assorted desks faced the blackboard in a long uneven row. There were two tables, and, next the fire, a high counting-house desk sacred to the headmaster. This room served as our common-room as well as classroom. Most of our waking hours were spent in it.

Not long after supper I was taken to the dormitory to which I had been assigned. There were five beds in it; lights out was at 8 p.m.

Like the dining-room, the dormitory was in the house itself; and as I discovered the next morning, looked out over a tennis-lawn bordered by hedges of yew and rhododendron. Hidden behind one of the hedges ran the Cliftonville Road, and beyond that, veget-able allotments straggled down the hill to Midsummer Meadow where the river Nen made a sluggish entry into the town to receive a donation of processed sewage and chemical waste. None of this could be seen from the dormitory windows except for two enor-mous cooling-towers. But though invisible, the mephitic purlieus of a decaying industrial town made themselves felt. For all that the school stood on high ground, a peculiar clotting stink – a com-bination of the smell of gasworks and the unmistakable pong of tanneries – clung round the place. On my first morning the twin cooling-towers were just discernible from the dormitory window; pure shapes of pearly colour shimmering behind a gauze of dank, immobile yellow fog – the standard fare of a winter's day at Northampton in the thirties.

Six

The deaf man is confined to the circumstances of
light, distance, posture of body, both in himself
and him he communicates with.

GEORGE DALGARNO, *Didascalocophus*

EVERY morning the school assembled for breakfast in the dining-
room. Two tables, an upper and a lower, accommodated the
twenty-odd pupils, the staff, the headmaster and his family. The
lower table was ruled by Miss Whittaker, a young woman who
taught the juniors and also took some of the senior boys for
French. Mr Ince-Jones, his wife, and two small daughters sat at the
head of the upper table. At its other end the matron, Miss Castles,
poured tea and kept order. The pupils were distributed haphazard,
changing places and tables once a week. There was good reason
for this: the system ensured that three or four times a term each
boy was brought into informal quasi-social daily contact with the
headmaster. It was part of our education.

Breakfast over, we returned to the large schoolroom in the outbuildings. The four prefects then saw to it that each of us, in hier-
archical order, visited one of the two outside lavatories, there to
perform the first duty of the day.

This exercise would be followed by prayers at 9.15. The school
stood to attention until the headmaster stalked in, black-gowned,
magisterial. He would recite the Lord's Prayer which we repeated
after him line by line. Next, if there were occasion, we would
listen to whatever decree or fiat the headmaster desired to add to
the elaborate accretion of laws and taboos that we were required
to observe. Or to a brief but ominous homily on our collective
moral shortcomings. Or one miserable offender might be singled
out to have expounded the inherent evil of his nature and doings;
with a brimstone whiff of the wrath to come. At least once a
term the headmaster blew us all up, *en masse* and individually.
The cause of this detonation was always the same: the wearing or
rather non-wearing of the school tie, an inoffensive affair of plain

green wool or cotton. The headmaster might begin by observing that the senior prefect, who should be setting an example to one and all, was disgracing his responsible office by omitting to don the regulation neckwear. He would then work down through the rest of the school, find nobody in a green tie, and from there work up to a peroration which left us shaking in our shoes. Next day and for a week thereafter all would turn out in uniform ties; then motley would creep back. For as a school we had, thank God, no real esprit de corps but remained individuals.

Immediately after prayers a screen was put up to divide the senior class, taken by the headmaster, from Mr Mundin's junior class at the more temperate end of the room. The infants and the very backward were looked after by Miss Whittaker in a small separate classroom at the other side of the building.

All teaching was by the spoken word: we were expected to lip-read (and did) every syllable uttered in class. The method of instruction cannot have differed much from that practised in hearing schools, apart from the immense pains taken to elucidate each subject. The substance of every sentence might be repeated over and over again, each time in a slightly different way, until the dullest had grasped the point. It would then be written down on the blackboard, a brick in the little edifice of information painstakingly being constructed for us. Then the next point would be taken up, clarified, and added to the remarks already on the board. By the end of the lesson a brief essay would have been chalked up, which we were then required to copy into our exercise books – ready-made notes of the lecture, as it were.

These repetitions of the major points in the lesson sometimes sent me daydreaming even while I lipread. The headmaster or Mr Mundin, or whoever was teaching, would sometimes stop in mid-sentence if he suspected a boy's attention to be wandering, point an imperative and interrogatory finger at the offender and oblige him to prove he had been following the lesson by repeating what had just been said. At these times my thoughts might be far away and I would have no more idea of what I had been lipreading than the man in the moon. Yet I was generally able to parrot back the teacher's last dozen words, without really having a notion what they were – often I listened with interest to myself repeating them. I had developed a knack for lipreading without taking in the message, a reprehensible accomplishment. No one ever tumbled to the fact that because I could echo what had been said word for word, it did not follow that I had been 'listening'. I offer the phenomenon to the non-deaf reader as a curiosity; doubtless he has had the same experience in auditory terms.

Noise was the only unusual feature of these classes. I should explain that the ordinary method of demanding attention from a pupil (especially if he happened not to be looking) was a thump of the magisterial heel. This could be heard reverberating through the floorboards even by those who like me were deafer than the grave. Behind the screen Mr Mundin would be requiring attention from members of his own class by similar stampings – yet we could easily distinguish between his deferentially toned-down heel-thud and the eruption, as of the grounding of a thunderbolt, which emanated from the headmaster.

Sometimes the latter might be taking two classes simultaneously – one standing up for questions and answers, the other doing desk-work. The heel-thuds directed at the standing class did not disturb the desk-workers even when emphatic enough to shake ink from the inkwells. But did the headmaster require the attention of any one of the desk-workers he would aim, so to speak, a tattoo in his direction and that boy would know it was for him. I don't know how it was done, I can only affirm the fact – for many a time I would be unconcernedly reading or writing throughout a thunderous session and suddenly, with an electric jolt to my heart, pick out and obey the unmistakable imperative thump directed at myself.

The day always began with the noisiest lesson – arithmetic. Six or seven of us stood in an apprehensive half-circle while problems in mental arithmetic were fired at us – simple sums to start with, of the there-are-five-apples-in-a-basket-Joe-eats-two-how-many-are-left type, followed by progressively harder ones involving fractions and decimal places. We dreaded the arithmetic period. The brains of deaf-born boys work slowly – inadequate grasp of language has to do with this – and can get locked for minutes on end in what seems monumental stupidity. At such times the strain of years of continuous teaching of the deaf might begin to tell and on a bad day one of these arithmetic classes could wind up in a paroxysm of heel-hammering and repeated bellowings – 'How many? How many?' – at the morning's dunce, by now reduced to a pulp of terror, the functioning of his mental machinery effectively stalled. The din could be unbelievable.

The elaborate repetition and clarification of each point which was a feature of our lessons at Northampton often made me feel impatient, though it helped to fix them almost effortlessly in my memory. I had a greater range of general information than most of the others – about the average for a boy of my age – because unlike them I could and did read for pleasure.* But it is almost impossible to exaggerate the narrow scope of the general information of a deaf-born boy whose vocabulary may sometimes be too scanty to allow him to browse over a popular newspaper. This cuts him off from one main source of spontaneous self-instruction; the other, common every-day talk with people, is inhibited; and the radio is of course no use to him. Nowadays there is the telly which no doubt makes a difference, but in those days it did not exist. If knowledge be compared to light, most hearing people live in a twilight precinct with one or two brightly lit patches – subjects with which they have special acquaintance. But my companions, it seemed to me, existed in a pitchblackness shot through with a few concentrated beams of painfully gathered information. Thus in the course of almost every lesson some basic piece of enlightenment had to be imparted to one or other of the class who turned out to be ignorant of some fact which most people would assume was generally known – to give an extreme example, that hens lay eggs. Of course we were not as absolutely ignorant as this might imply – but each of us had different areas of total unawareness of elementary facts. For this reason the headmaster instituted a daily class in reading the newspapers. And he and the rest of the staff made it their business to use every minute of the time spent with us to pierce the carapace of ignorance that deafness entails.

For example our Wednesday half-holidays when, except in the case of really bad weather, we took a prescriptive bicycle outing under the wing of the headmaster. The senior boys were licensed,

* Though before I left Northampton Mr Mundin organized a lending library (the books being loaned each term by Northampton Public Library) and instituted a 'reading hour', I was one of the very few pupils who read to please himself. Apart from comics, the others seemed only to read when they were told, or for information about some hobby like stamp-collecting or fretwork. This was because a comparatively small vocabulary makes reading a painful process – exactly as when one reads a book in some half-assimilated foreign language for which the dictionary must be ever at hand. It was a vicious circle, for the less they read the less chance they gave themselves of expanding their vocabularies.

indeed enjoined, to own bicycles – rusty secondhand machines bought for a pound or two at the nearest cycle-repair shop. (As we were seldom allowed outside the school precincts we had not much use for them except on Wednesdays.) Punctually at two-thirty on those afternoons our cavalcade emerged from the school gates, riding in single file in a strict order of precedence. The head-master led, followed by the newest recruit to the bicycle corps, and thence in ascending order of recruitment or status, so that the most experienced riders brought up the rear. For these excursions the headmaster invariably clad himself in a suit of light blue plus-fours, khaki raincoat, old soft trilby hat and a black briar pipe. He rode an ancient and singular machine, high-saddled and somehow reminiscent of a middle-aged dromedary. Like all his possessions this bicycle was permeated by its owner's personality – an Ed-wardian solidity and stateliness that dispensed with mere elegance. All the headmaster's accessories – Homburg hats, silver-topped malacca, powderblue overcoat, and even so conveyor-belt an item as his Morris Oxford saloon car – were deeply impressed with his signature and might have been his appendages rather than belong-ings. That bicycle in particular seemed less a possession than an extension of the headmaster; who at that time was in his middle fifties, and, like Chaucer's Monk, no pale and wasting ghost. For him those weekly rides must have been something of an effort. Not only physically: for he made them serve an educational as well as a recreational purpose. Looking back I begin to appreciate the obsessive energy that he brought to his never-ending work of in-sinuating knowledge through the tough hide of our deafness. Every moment he was with us he was on the job, not least on these bicycle rides.

We didn't often do more than twenty miles in an afternoon and usually returned in time for tea. During my five years at Northampton we must have visited every village and church in-side a radius of ten miles. In spring we would be taken to Whittle-bury woods to admire metallic sheets of bluebells glinting through the undergrowth. Summer rides often led in the direction of Over-stone Park where we swam or mini-golfed. Winter found us visiting derelict Georgian mansions and decaying Victorian demi-palazzos, country houses that had been up for sale for decades. Older destinations included a country crematorium, and a private aerodrome at Sywell where we spent afternoons watching mous-tachioed youths – the Battle of Britain less than five years off –

learning to fly pocket biplanes which even then wore a period look. And invariably, when we reached our objective, or if the headmaster saw anything of interest on the way and decided to halt, he would signal us to dismount and thereupon, in the middle of a half-moon of attentively inattentive adolescents, patiently impart information – botanic, architectural, linguistic, agricultural, historical, social, cultural, political, animal, vegetable, mineral.

It was the headmaster's custom to eat *en famille* with his pupils. Our education never stopped so far as he was concerned. Luncheons he devoted to the attempt to introduce us to the art of conversation. Apart from his persevering opportunism in the matter of adding to our stock of general knowledge, he was concerned to get the ball of conversation going to and fro across the table – a far harder task than may seem to those who have no experience of the meagre verbal capacity of so many of the deaf-born. He was himself a good conversationalist, told a story well, and drew from a wide experience of places and people. For every summer he made a grand tour of Europe, where he hobnobbed with princes and politicians (that was my impression, but perhaps he had merely a weakness for name-dropping). His outlook may have been reactionary but was by no means provincial.

The school was dominated by his personality. He fascinated us, as a snake rabbits. He could charm the birds off the trees. He could also make them drop dead with fright. Recalling him now, with infinitely more knowledge and experience of people and the world than I had then, I realize that he was a truly remarkable man; also an actor, a superb actor. He had a magnificent profile, imposing forehead, large grey-green eyes set wide apart; features which bore an uncommon affinity to the patrician good looks of Sir Austen Chamberlain. Perhaps he cultivated the resemblance by wearing that eyeglass. His wife was an Irishwoman of great charm, a good deal younger than himself. The headmaster had been called to the bar as a young man, and if he had chosen to pursue the profession of barrister he would, I suspect, have made a fortune as an advocate. All the best barristers are born actors. He was very able; I never discovered why he had not followed a profession which he could have made so lucrative, to take up one so obscure as the teaching of the deaf. It was not an obvious vocation. But he had, if not what's called a social conscience, a strong sense of duty. Late in life, when he was about forty I think, he was confirmed to the Church of England – a late conversion somehow makes a man's religious conviction seem more serious.

To the assistant master of the school, E. L. Mundin, attached less panache; but perhaps he was overshadowed by the more spectacular personality. Slight, very dark, very neat, almost dapper, Mr Mundin radiated a kind of spare efficiency – all his movements were rapid, frugal, but precise. He taught us history and geography, took us for drill, football, and cricket, and on Saturday afternoons oversaw the entire school at carpentry. We had a well-equipped workshop converted from what must once have been a coach-house next the old stables, now the schoolroom. Some of us he turned into skilled carpenters; at least one of his pupils became, later, a professional woodcarver. At that time, before his marriage, Mr Mundin lived with his father, who was a well-known cabinet-maker in Northampton. From his father Mr Mundin inherited – and to some extent I caught from him – a peculiarly reverential attitude to tools and craftsmanship, an appreciation of the grain and quality of good wood and well-made furniture. (This appreciation has nothing to do with the aesthetic aspect, nor does the fact I have never been any use as a carpenter affect it.) When I arrived Mr Mundin was a young man, perhaps not quite thirty. He had been teaching at Northampton for over a dozen years. We looked upon him as the headmaster's heir-apparent, and so he might have been, but things did not work out in that way.

Like most teachers of the deaf, the headmaster and Mr Mundin spoke exceptionally well from the point of view of a lipreader. They never exaggerated lip movements – clear, precise, and above all natural pronunciation is the secret. But they would modify the speed to suit occasion – when delivering a general address they spoke at a slower tempo than when talking to one or two of the boys. If they wanted to say something privately to each other without being 'overheard' they used to rattle off the words between almost closed teeth, far too fast to be picked up by the best of us.

All instruction and communication at the school was entirely oral so far as the headmaster and staff were concerned. We were spoken to in the ordinary way, with no resort whatever to signs or gestures (our manner of talking with each other, the 'sign-language' or argot I have described, was of course strictly prohibited – 'signing' was a punishable offence). If a word were not understood, it was not written down but repeated. The only classes I can recall that would not have been included in the curriculum of an ordinary school were the speech classes, the newspaper-reading class, and a class for practising speech and hearing with the aid of a big amplifier with headphones. There were no lipreading classes as such, for in a sense all lessons were lipreading lessons. A few tips on lipreading would be passed on from time to time, for example how to distinguish – as far as they may be distinguished – those three hardy identicals, P, B, and M, how to look out for the slight trembling of the nose that shows that N rather than T or D is being said.

Concerning the art, craft, or skill of lipreading a few points may here be made. I never 'learnt' to lipread, it came to me naturally – as it does to people who work in noisy factories and can hardly tell whether they hear or lipread what is said to them. But lipreading is not simply a physical operation in which the eye has learnt to interpret for the ear, it is also an intellectual exercise. Lipreading is ninety per cent guesswork, because while most vowels are easily distinguished many consonants are not, since these are often produced by nearly identical lip movements. This means that in effect a great number of words and syllables which are distinct in sound appear to the eye as like as peas. Here is an example of half a dozen words sharing the same vowel, and for the lipreader practically indistinguishable one from the other: *mat, mad, bat, bad, pat,* and *pad* (P, B and M again). When any of these comes up the lipreader has to guess which of the six it may be; the syntax or context of the phrase or sentence in which it occurs will give a clue, and so will the general subject of the conversation. The alternatives can be so many that it may take a lipreader a few seconds to make the choice while he runs the various possibilities through his mind.* Sometimes he has to 'play back' a phrase or sentence more than once, revisualizing the lip movements with his inner eye (as it might be a film sequence run through again and again on a cutting-room projector), till there is a quite appreciable time gap between the eye's reception of a word

* I may as well give here a famous trap sentence used by Alexander Graham Bell, the inventor of the telephone, to demonstrate the ambiguities of speech when read by the eye. He would say, 'It rate ferry aren't hadn't four that reason high knit donned co.' The lipreader would repeat what he thought he had seen Bell say: 'It rained very hard and for that reason I did not go.'

and the mind's interpretation or reading of it. All the while, the lipreader's eye is engaged in taking the next sentence or two, and at the same time he is working out a reply or rejoinder to keep his end of the conversation going. This sort of triple exercise can be fatiguing. People differ, but as I grow older I find an hour or two's solitude every day (or just being somewhere where no one is going to talk to me) a necessity.

There are of course words which for one reason or another are less easy to read than others. What happens, then, is that in practice lipreading becomes a joint operation shared by the lipreader and his interlocutor. For the interlocutor takes part in rendering his communication intelligible. He not only takes trouble to speak clearly and slowly, but exercises a deliberate and selective choice of vocabulary – avoiding, for instance, words he guesses or knows from experience to be ambiguous or difficult for the other to read. This labour of communicating influences the *kind* of conversation offered to the deaf. When speaking to a lipreader people naturally get into the habit of expressing themselves with greater directness and concision; to come to the nub of what they have to say with less waffling around the bush. So it comes about that the deaf (or such is my impression) are asked to submit to less meaningless chat for the sake of chat than most people. In their case conversation remains more of a vehicle of entertainment and exchange of ideas than it is for many people who use talk as a device to caulk the interstices of silence; not really listening but needing it as a comforting background noise, like radio or gramophone.

At the age of fourteen people are usually unhappy. So was I. Not on account of the emotional problems of adolescence (that was for later) but because of the radical change of environment, of place and people. The skies of England, everlastingly lidded with soggy clouds; an infinite repetition of sootgrained streets; perpetual invisibility of sun, moon, and stars; and, in what passed for 'the country', cabined fields constricted by hedgerows and tarmac roads – all these cumbered and dejected my spirits. But most clogging of all, until I adjusted to it, was life at school.

After the freedom of the South African day-school I felt as if thrust into a straitjacket. The Northampton school seemed governed by an intricate accretion of rules and prohibitions (mostly prohibitions). Yet they were probably no more numerous or stringent than those of many other English boarding-schools. Most of all I disliked the rule forbidding us to leave the school unescorted, except for a couple of hours on Saturday mornings. Another prescript ensured the censorship of outgoing letters. These, whether to parents or friends or the manufacturers of bodybuilding harness, had to be submitted to the headmaster before posting. It was explained that this would ensure they contained no mistakes of grammar or spelling (and to be fair the syntax and orthography of some of us bordered on the surrealistic). There remained the invasion of privacy, particularly the overseeing of relationships with parents. We countered by writing letters composed of unexceptionable sentiments tagged to a bald summary of events. These were the two restrictions that irked most. But what I found exasperating and dreary was the cumulative effect of the maze of petty fiats and 'not alloweds'.

The network of taboos and vetoes was not wholly the doing of 'them' – the headmaster and staff – but in great part of the boys themselves. This may have been a reflection of English puritanism – its delight in abnegation and interdict.* The examples I could give are piddling, which is the point. Innovations or exhibitions of personal initiative were nearly always disapproved of and where possible forbidden. On our prefect-escorted Sunday walks inane prohibitions used to be invented on the spot. I remember a dog coming up to me in the park – I bent to pat it on the head. 'Not allowed!' cries one of my companions, nudging me aside and shooing the dog off. At the top of the Little Billing Road we used to pass a Walls stop-me-and-buy-one ice-cream tricycle (now there's a period piece), but the notion that any of us should, like the free citizens all around, stop it and buy one, would be received with moral indignation. Not allowed! It might have been the school slogan. Years later when I became a prefect in course of time, and had authority to combat this kind of pointless self-mortification, I discovered by asking the headmaster that there was in fact no such prohibition. As I might have guessed. But when I gave my charges permission to buy ice-cream if they wished, it was regarded as being in some way morally subversive.

* You can see it today in the satisfaction with which you are told you can't buy a drink, or have something to eat, or whatever it may be; in the enthusiasm with which British Railways and the tube trains have jumped at the chance of turning three-quarters of their carriages into non-smokers, on the excuse of combating lung-cancer.

For the first couple of terms the headmaster and staff gave me a fairly rough time. They were breaking me in. Later I was to see other newcomers undergoing the same purgatory. It was probably necessary. Deaf children can be badly spoiled by parents who subconsciously feel, as so many do, that somehow the child's disability is their fault. In trying to make up for it they let him have his own way too easily and often. This is aided and abetted by friends and relations who cannot help feeling sorry for the child. The end-product is often an intensely selfish and unattractive infant. To counteract intensive spoiling, new boys went through a disciplinary crash course.

At my hearing school I had hardly ever been punished, not that I remember doing anything particularly heinous. None the less, consciously or unconsciously I was becoming used to exceptions being made in my favour; to me the benefit of the doubt had been extended often enough for me to look on it as an inalienable right. Not overtly but in fact my status was that of an object of pity. At Northampton I lost the advantage of my disadvantage: my deafness was useless, the others were deaf too. I learned one good lesson: I was not the only cracked pebble on the beach. As will be seen, I do not think the deaf should have too much to do with each other; yet it is only the deaf who can teach the deaf how to live without trading on deafness. Among hearing people it is too easy, often too much of a temptation, for the deaf child to deal in their pity and guilt, or charity and kindness, till the plain truth that nobody owes him anything because he cannot hear is mislaid or never learned; to be painfully rediscovered when he grows up.

From the beginning the headmaster set out to demonstrate that I could not get away with anything whatever. At the slightest insubordination (even if unintentional as often it was while I threaded a path through the labyrinth of regulations which ordered every detail of the day) down he came like a cartload of bricks. So long as I was the school's latest recruit he had his eye on me – a monocled, terrible eye; a step wrong, a least failure of submission or courtesy, and that histrionic brow darkened, lightning flashed and the sky reverberated. Against me he never lifted a hand; perhaps I should have been less frightened if he had.

The usual punishment was lines – fifty, a hundred, two hundred, anything up to a thousand reiterations of some nugatory exhortation. In my first year I don't think there could have been a day when I wasn't working off my backlog, scribbling, scribbling, in the breaks, after prep, and in the hour before bed. It ate (as intended) into the scraps of spare time I had for reading, and it ruined (as presumably not intended) my handwriting. After I left school I scarcely took up a pen again except to sign my name – even to compose poems I use a typewriter.

The pressure came off after the first couple of terms. Another new boy arrived, to be put through the same mangle. I began to settle down and even to enjoy myself.

At first, as a deaf boy among deaf boys, I felt far more of a fish out of water than ever I did at my hearing school. It was not that I could find no friends; but that rapport was inhibited by limitations of vocabulary and experience. We were not on the same wavelength; it took time for me to tune in. But Northampton had one advantage, not to be sneezed at, over my South African preparatory school. There was no bullying. The usual modes of schoolboy torture were unheard of. Hardly any violence took place among us. I recall no fights, above all no physical cruelty, though once I was nearly knocked out by a blow to the head delivered with full force by a seventeen-year-old giant. But there was no malice behind it and I did not mind. The boy who hit me, despite his age and size, counted as one of the 'juniors'; he could hardly speak or write. He had long arms and powerful muscles but difficulty in coordinating their movements; and he had no idea of his own strength. Besides I had been annoying him and had made him lose his temper.

The deaf don't often lose their tempers, but when they do it can be catastrophic. On this matter I speak subjectively. Berserk is hardly the word for what happens: every vein seems filled with sheetlightning. For myself I become totally unable to lipread or to understand any kind of communication till the paroxysm is over. It is a form of possession, and at its apex the rage is no longer directed at whatever may have been the immediate provocation but at the whole incommunicable uncommunicating universe; as if every minor inconvenience and thread of suffering had been woven into a single unbearable explosive bundle; it is at deafness one rages. So when angry I have to be careful – careful not to let myself go in case I go too far. This has done me out of not a few satisfying lettings-off of steam. Other deaf men, I believe, are in the same case; which may explain why so many of them are usually gentle and even-tempered, or seem to be.

On Sundays the school was one of the famous sights of Northampton. This was the day we appeared in a uniform of dark serge suits, black ties, black shoes, starched collars and bowler hats. (In summer we exchanged bowlers for straw boaters. I don't know which we hated worse.) Getting the studs fixed into a stiff collar and then turning down the intractable material over one's tie is a fiendish job, especially on a grating midwinter morning. In this rig, archaic even for the thirties, we assemble in the schoolroom half an hour before church. The prefects make an inspection; bowlers have to be rebrushed and specks of dirt massaged off, or into, blue serge suits. Then, rawchinned and bowlerhatted, we march two by two in a long crocodile up the Billing Road past the general hospital and rococo town hall to make our entry into the church by the side door of the south aisle. It is a large Wren-style church of the kind appropriate to a solid provincial market town. In it, ours is a gallingly conspicuous position. Not for us the decent obscurity of the pewboxes: our allotted place is a long column of chairs, two abreast, set in the middle of the central aisle. The vicar and choir file past us on either side on their way to the altar; then the long ennui of a ceremony we can neither hear nor take part in begins.

Until I hit on the idea of whiling time away by plugging through the Bible from one end to the other, the services seemed unending – particularly on those black Sundays when they embarked on the Litany. The only entertainment would be provided by the sermon.

Its preacher, a magnanimous unselfconscious cleric, was in fact a famous orator. As our parish priest he used to visit the school at least once a term; we loved him. We also loved to watch him preach. Huge and unwieldy, the tattered fringe of his black gown flapping slowly behind him, he would mount the carved oak pulpit. As he gave the text of his sermon he looked exactly like a weatherbeaten old shellback in the crow's-nest of a sailing-ship. Imperceptibly at first but with mounting tempo as his discourse gathered momentum, he would begin to roll and sway from one side to another. Not gently swaying but lurching, staggering, while he gripped the pulpit rail till knuckles shone white in the stained-glass gloom. He might really have been in the crosstrees of a schooner beating up the channel in half a gale. Yet all he was doing was to try to balance his enormous body on the outside edges of the soles of his boots. (We had deduced this from observing him at the lectern, where feet were visible.) Lost in his sermon, for minutes on end he would manage his balancing act, rhythmically teetering, until one of the boot soles slipped and he would either pitch forward or starkly subside as if about to disappear through a trapdoor. He and his congregation, rapt in his extempore address, appeared completely oblivious of these oscillations, which indeed conveyed – or is this my fancy? – something of its fervour to us, the watchers.

Sunday afternoons were dedicated to walks – the smaller boys under the escort of one of the staff. But the dozen or so seniors divided themselves among the four prefects, each of whom led a cohort of two or three on whatever promenade took his fancy. Gloved and bowlerhatted, the parties set off on vague perambulations round the town, or towards the few reachable patches of countryside. Usually we avoided Abingdon Park and similar public resorts. We were known by our conspicuous Sunday garb: witty urchins too often were tempted to entertain themselves and their friends by mounting derisory parodies of the deaf-and-dumb finger-alphabet when they spotted our approach. Our favourite haunt was the canal, behind the gasworks. A wasteland of derelict back-streets enlivened by tobacconist-newsagent corner-shops behind whose flyblown panes dummy cigarette-packets, disposed in sagging pyramids, provide a background for grit-covered copies of *Gem*, *Magnet*, *Wizard*, and *Rover*, for jars of deliquescing bullseyes, dusty sticks of black liquorice in foxed and fading wrappers, short clay pipes with bowls moulded in the likeness of Gladstone or General Gordon. This area debouches upon a yet forlorner wilderness through which slides the canal, its towing-path fenced by high, rusting, blackpainted sheets of corrugated iron garnished with festering strands of barbed wire. A railway bridge straddles the water. Here we wait for the London express to trail a glittering ribbon over the fetidities; which event furnishes the climax of that particular walk. Another promenade fetches us to Eleanor's Cross on the outskirts of Northampton, via the old battlefield near the sewage farm and the village of Hardingstone. Outside Hardingstone a blackened chassis on the grass verge is pointed out as the remains of the car in which the salesman-Lothario Alfred Rouse burned the murdered body of a tramp in the hope it might be taken for his own. Not all walks were like these; in summer, particularly early summer, we could wander by alluvial meadows alongside the river Nen, gold sheets of buttercups bordered by green hedgerows. Here we would look for and sometimes find the nests of lapwings; for Northampton still has, or had, its ruralities. The town may have been grim, but its griminess was besieged by the most beautiful of the midland shires.

One of the singular features of the school was the stretch of its corporate memory. Like the tribal chroniclers of the Zulus we had no written records but maintained a kind of oral history. The repositories of this history were those boys who had been at school longest (in my time one of them had been there more than a decade, having come when he was seven and stayed till he was well over twenty). Thus I came to hear, in time, the biography of practically every pupil who had attended the school, some of whom must have left it ten or even twenty years before my arrival. Their characters, idiosyncracies, their very appearance were kept alive by partly mimed reconstructions of scandals and famous crises in which they had taken a part. In parenthesis, the best reportage I ever listened to (watched may be the word) came from my companions at Northampton. I even find it hard to remember whether I actually witnessed, or only heard about, some of the contretemps that occurred during my time at school, for any dramatic happening (we were inveterate gossips) would be immediately retailed for the benefit of those who had missed it – the narrator (or historian) reproducing the actions and mannerisms of each participant so graphically that the incidents seemed to take place before one's eyes. Years after I left school I met an ex-Northamptonian – a White Russian stage-designer and scene-painter – in a Soho pub. Though I had never met him before I not only knew all about him but recognized him on the spot (his beard, grown after he had left Northampton, had passed into school legend) and we were able to plunge at once into gossip about his contemporaries at the school, all of whom had preceded me there and few of whom I had in fact met, but with whose biographies I was perfectly familiar.

In the same way I heard a good deal about the school prodigy, who had left a couple of years before I arrived at Northampton. His career had been phenomenal – although his education proper had not begun until he came to Northampton when he was sixteen, a late age even for a deaf boy. When he arrived he was, so they told me, ignorant of simple arithmetic; yet a few years later had matriculated, entered London University, and gained a B.Sc. This had been achieved by a combination of brilliant coaching on one side and gargantuan application on the other. The boy never stopped working; sometimes he had had to be forbidden his books. The others admired, even more than his success, his colossal powers of concentration.

'Work, work, work,' the oral historian recites, awe on his face, rhythmically chopping the edge of his right hand into the heel of the other.

'Read, read, read,' the historian goes on; and creates a figure hunched over a desk with a book before him, hands shading the eyes to ward off distraction. Only once, it was related, had he failed an examination. The day before he sat for it he read in the paper that fish was good for the brain, bought two tins of sardines, conscientiously ate every last one of them, and was sick all night.

Twice or thrice I met him when he came to Northampton to play for the Old Boys in the annual cricket match. He had been one of the mainstays of the school eleven. In spite of poor vision (he wore pebble lenses) he was a remarkably successful bat. His batting was of a piece with his character – dogged, meticulous, unbelievably persevering. For every kind of ball, long hop, full toss, short length, good length, leg break, off break, he had one and the same stroke: a perfectly executed forward play in classic Victorian style. He never missed the ball and he broke the bowlers' hearts.

His university career was an uninterrupted success. First he collected his B.Sc.; and some years later a doctorate for a thesis on geology. No deaf-born man had equalled, and few have since surpassed, that academic record.

Another of my schoolfellows, Henry Garnet, comes back to me as one of the remarkable people I have known, though he could barely enunciate three intelligible words. Bowed like an elderly parrot, he spent every minute of his free time at his desk, either writing or reading. The subject of his studies was the royal family. From newspapers, illustrated weeklies and magazines he culled every reference to the king and queen and in particular the daughters of the duke and duchess of York. Their photographs he collected as they appeared day by day in the public prints. When he was not reading about the royal family he was scribbling page after page of jumbled English, words following one another with

71

little syntactical relation, a sort of dream-language evolved from the columns of newsprint on which he browsed. No sentence could be understood by itself but the subject was plain: the royal family. He could have been Smike at Dotheboys Hall, writing endless letters to the duke of Wellington. But Henry Garnet wrote his text in vertical columns like a newspaper's; these were inset, in lieu of photographs, with painstaking crayon drawings. Now and then he would get out his paints and provide a sumptuous coloured supplement, invariably a large-scale portrait of one or more of his royal personages. He preferred to depict his king and queen in full regalia – crowns, orbs, sceptres, and ermines; with backgrounds of more than imperial splendour – thrones, hangings, attendant flunkeys, gold-encrusted furniture. I now wish I had asked him to let me keep one of these paintings – after thirty years I still recall them with extraordinary distinctness. But at the time I thought them merely incompetent.

The father of one of the pupils, an international art-dealer of some kind, presented a silver cup for the best original painting by a pupil of the school. This aroused any amount of excitement, for every one of the boys (myself the miserable exception) had a more than average ability in draughtsmanship. Many elaborate projects were embarked on, and a whole term devoted to their completion. Before the paintings were handed in we agreed that the prize would probably go to one of the prefects, who had offered a perfectly executed chocolate-box painting of a Spanish treasure-galleon. It was flamboyantly drawn and much admired. We were dumbfounded when the result was announced. The cup had gone to Henry Garnet. His offering – for him a routine picture, one of his portrait-groups of the royal family – had more originality and imagination to the square inch, remarked the art-dealer, than the rest of our paintings put together. Long afterwards I saw what he meant. Henry Garnet's pictures had something of the same quality I came to appreciate in the work of Alfred Wallis and the douanier Rousseau – the forcefulness of an obsessed imagination.

In my second year at Northampton I was entered for the Oxford Junior Local examination, more or less for a dummy run. To everyone's astonishment (mine too) I not only passed but passed with flying colours, owing to the good and careful tuition I received and to the fact I am one of those who have a knack for examinations, just as some people have a knack for crosswords. As I was no good at football, cricket, billiards, tennis, carpentry, drawing (what, will the list stretch to the crack of doom?) this improved my status – at least there was something I *could* do.

Apart from that I began to find much to enjoy, particularly the half-term holidays. Every summer, by tradition, we spent a June day playing cricket on the huge lawn below the lettered parapets and Jacobean façade of Inigo Jones's Castle Ashby; and there would be strawberries and cream. On the spring and autumn half-terms we took excursions into Northamptonshire, to Naseby, the middle point of England, with the hedged battlefield stretched beneath its church tower and the springs of Avon not far away; to Sulgrave, the manor belonging to forebears of Washington; and once to Canons Ashby, where the two Misses Dryden, of the same family as the poet, then still lived; its lawns and cedar remain part of my spiritual furniture. Somehow the sun always shone on those days.

In my first summer at Northampton I had difficulty getting to sleep. Lights out was at 8 p.m. – broad daylight in May or June. Having been brought up in a latitude where darkness never falls later than seven in the evening, I found it impossible to doze off while light remained in the sky. So I lay awake each evening waiting for the dark. As I could not read I began to amuse myself by repeating what poetry I remembered. This turned out to be a good way of passing the long, boring summer twilight, particularly as I could recite aloud without disturbing anybody. At first I could recall only fragments of poems. I got into the way of looking these up in the daytime, until I found I had a repertoire of half a dozen complete poems and any number of odd verses from a score of others. Without deliberately learning poems by heart (that would have been work, not fun) I reached the stage where I could give a recitation lasting over an hour, without repeating a single item. Nearly all these poems came from the *Oxford Book of English Verse*. Most of the Shakespeare sonnets in that anthology became part of my repertoire. But my star turn, which took several weeks to perfect, was the whole of *Lycidas*. This poem I cannot have more than half understood, in the sense that I had any notion where Deva was or who sage Hippotades might be. It was a case of the operation of Eliot's Law: in poetry communication precedes understanding. As far as enjoyment goes I began positively looking forward to lights out, that I might set going what seemed to me marvellous harmonies – in the case of Milton, harmonies made reverberant by the romantic and imposing proper names dispensed in the verse:

> Whilst the the shores, and sounding Seas
> Wash far away, where ere thy bones are hurld,
> Whether beyond the stormy *Hebrides*,
> Where thou perhaps under the whelming tide
> Visit'st the bottom of the monstrous world;
> Or whether thou to our moist vows deny'd,
> Sleep'st by the fable of *Bellerus* old,
> Where the great vision of the guarded Mount
> Looks toward *Namancos* and *Bayona's* hold,
> Look homeward Angel now, and melt with ruth.
> And, O ye Dolphins, waft the hapless youth.

Lying in bed I watched twilight thicken while in the soundbox of my head I listened to my own voice perform a private concert. For poetry attracted me as music, what Dryden called 'articulate music'. I did not speak the poems: I chanted and declaimed, pulling out the stops of sound, rapt in the unrolling of rhythm and images. Anything onomatopoeic I was a pushover for, especially if the verse were an attempt to imitate the sound of musical instruments: Milton's *Blest Pair of Sirens*, Dryden's *Ode on St Cecilia's Day*, Browning's *A Toccata of Gallupi's*, and the bit about the bells in *High Tide on the Coast of Lincolnshire*. Most of my adolescence coincided not unnaturally with a passion for sonorously nostalgic stuff like Tennyson's *Lotus Eaters* and Rossetti's *Blessed Damozel*. I was not above Kipling; and somehow got on to Donne:

> Since I am comming to that Holy roome,
> Where, with thy Quire of Saints for evermore,
> I shall be made thy Musique; As I come,
> I tune the Instrument here at the dore . . .

After *Lycidas* I should think my favourite recitativo was Browning's *Waring*, for much the same reason: the shiftings of pace and rhythm, the orchestration, the rum and exotic images – a Czar garotted in the Kremlin, the bloody head of Orpheus rolled along a torrent.

Had anyone heard me it must have sounded like a horrible

droning chant. Yet these nightly concerts were probably the best training I could have given myself in metric and the handling of vowels and consonants, in the relations of sense and sound, in the orchestration of a poem. My habit has always been, then and now, to listen to the noise a poem makes before beginning to attend to what it is actually saying or projecting. The auditory rather than the visual captures my imagination in the first place. I daresay it shouldn't.

While on the subject I may as well add that to begin with I found the metric of some poetry – quite apart from what used to be called 'modern', which at Northampton I barely met with – too subtle to appreciate. If I took pleasure in Shakespeare's sonnets it was long before his blank verse 'came across', and then it was the sugared beat he uses in *Romeo and Juliet*; I preferred Marlowe's mighty line, or mighty thump. It was a good while before my ear had been educated enough to appreciate the contrapuntal effects in *Lear*. In the same way the blank verse of *Paradise Lost* eluded me, though, seduced as I had been by *Lycidas*, I tried again and again. Then one day – I must have been about sixteen – all at once I got it, as if the lines had lifted trumpets to their mouths. *Samson Agonistes* held out a bit longer.

More than once the headmaster drove some of us to Stratford-on-Avon when the examination play was being performed. At the Memorial Theatre I saw *Julius Caesar* and *Twelfth Night*, though the production that sticks in my mind was a humbler but brilliantly staged version of *Macbeth* at the Northampton Repertory Theatre, whose designer, Osborne Robinson, was already famous. With Shakespeare, if one knew the play well (as we certainly did in the case of set plays) it was easy to follow almost every word spoken by the actors.

Summer was always a good term. Every other week we had a cricket match with one of the hearing schools. We could give a good account of ourselves too: the local grammar school, with 600 pupils to draw from, hated to lose to us, and always had a run for its money. This match, the most important of the season, was generally played on a ground almost as fabulous as the park of Castle Ashby: a field belonging to the Northampton Lunatic Asylum.* It overlooked the Nen, a green carpet suspended above

* The same asylum that sheltered John Clare for nearly a quarter of a century.

the river valley. We visited the county cricket ground often – sometimes for the whole day when the Australians or South Africans were playing. Though no good as a player I became an addict, and on this ground saw most of the already legendary figures of the thirties – Hammond, Larwood, Bradman, Sutcliffe, Hendren, Bowes and Verity.

Yes, we had good times; but cabined, cribbed, confined, bound in – for only once a week were we allowed out of the school gates. This was on Saturday mornings, when for a couple of hours we had the freedom of the town to do our shopping. (We got sixpence a week pocket-money; it now seems incredible what that could buy.) For the rest of the week we were prisoners. It seems that authority had never recovered from a traumatic event which took place in some remote era, probably before most of us were born, and which, it appeared, accounted for the convent-like restrictions placed upon us. One of the pupils had succeeded in putting a local girl in the family way.

'The filthy beast!' authority would comment, as it recounted the abomination with flashing eye and curling upper lip.

The reaction evoked in us by this anecdote might have surprised authority: a complex of awe, envy, wild surmise and wilder hope. Why, none of us would have dared to *speak* to a girl, let alone . . .

Mount Athos might have been the model, the way temptation was exiled from us. Of the school's two maids, one, poor woman, had a hare-lip; no more monumentally devenustated a female ever trod. As for the other, we seemed to have a new one every term – perhaps because it was impossible to find a servant-girl who did not appear as aphrodite beside the ineffable disfigurement of the first. All that could be done was done to stamp out sex. Midnight forays into dormitories and sudden switchings-on of lights now and then resulted in a revelation of scandalous juxta-positionings. Of the deleterious effects of these activities, including masturbation, we were kept fully informed. But it and they went on; the big stick was wielded, but in vain.

Holidays I spent with my mother and her sister at Liverpool. My aunt Mat had apartments at the top of a cadaverous Victorian house in Croxteth Road at the edge of Prince's Park. It seemed scarcely less a prison than Northampton. In the thirties Liverpool stood plutonian and overpowering, an apparently everlasting monument to the industrial revolution. They have now scraped away the grime, but I am glad to have seen St George's Hall in its ebony patina, stark against a gunmetal sky weeping tears of soot; to have known those rhadamanthine avenues of sable masonry. down which so many tramcars, dense with passengers as blackly clad as their city, shouldered along wheelbright rails from murk to murk. Oppressive, ponderous, weighing on the imagination, Liverpool at least had the grandeur of an extreme.

At Liverpool began a battle which lasted through adolescence. It was one that is probably fought by many deaf children: against overprotective love. A deaf and only child stands in double danger of the possessive element in maternal love – at least one deaf boy I knew became his mother's prisoner, his initiative and identity so atrophied by that protecting care that as himself he seemed scarcely to exist. My peril was nothing like as extreme, for my mother remained essentially a down-to-earth Scotswoman full of the practical common sense that might be expected of her peasant stock. Yet where I was concerned these admirable qualities sometimes ceased to operate. This was understandable but a great pity, for it infected our relationship. The accident of my deafness had been a traumatic experience for my mother. As a consequence much of my adolescence was determined by the need to escape from the maternal neurosis.

Until I came to England I had been free to go where I wished, at least in the suburbs of Johannesburg where we lived. If I went to the city centre, it would be with one of my parents or a school friend. At the Liverpool flat it was different. The heavy city traffic terrified my mother. She ˙as convinced that I was bound to be run over if I tried to cross the road on my own. She forbade me to leave the house without an escort – which in effect meant under the wing of my aunt or mother or both. But I could not take the perpetual detention which seemed to have become my lot since I landed in England: nine months of the year locked up at school, the remainder kennelled in a Liverpool flat. So one morning I slipped out of the house and took a short constitutional up a couple of terraced streets. Apprehensive of my mother's anxiety I came back within a quarter of an hour. Things were much as I feared on my return: my mother collapsed on a sofa, my aunt distraught. Hands were for wringing and tears came by the bucket: all the stops of feminine blackmail well and truly pulled out.

I hardened my heart, realizing it was her or me. Next day I

made a similar short excursion. There was another scene. But I persevered. The following morning I went out again. This time the repercussions rather lost edge for both of us.

Finding that I invariably returned undamaged, my mother reconciled herself to these perilous absences. By the end of a week I had won a tacit right to a brief morning perambulation on my own. Gradually I extended the length of my walks until it had been established that I was capable of looking after myself even in the face of city traffic.

It was the thin end of a wedge, as we both knew perfectly well. For the next year or two I devoted myself to widening it till I had got what I wanted: complete personal freedom. This I could only have obtained by cruelly subjecting my mother to anxiety – how else could I prove it was groundless? Later on, while spending a summer holiday in Scotland, I followed the same technique with a bicycle. At first I was allowed to cycle under escort (a laborious system which involved my mother riding in front, myself following; when she heard a car approaching from behind she would dismount and wait for it to pass; I was expected to do the same). There were heartrending scenes when I took to going off on short spins by myself. But by the time I was sixteen the battle was over; I could go out all day alone on a bicycle and not raise a qualm.

This compulsive anxiety was entirely concentrated on one thing: my deafness. My mother was not in the least bothered unless it were a question of my being at a disadvantage because I could not hear. She did not, for example, turn a hair when I took up rock-climbing in Arran one summer; even though I once fell thirty feet down a chimney on Cir Mhor. Years afterwards, during the war, I found myself piqued to discover that the prospect of a flying bomb alighting in my neighbourhood (I lived in London, my mother in the country) disquieted her a good deal less than it did me.

In the Oxford Junior Local examination I had come away with more 'honours', as good markings were then called, than any other candidate. This convinced me (as I hadn't expected even to pass in the first place) that I must have a flair for examinations. The next thing was to exploit it and go for the Oxford Senior Local. If you got a certain number of credits for that, you had matriculated; and if you matriculated, you could enter a university. At what stage the idea of getting into Oxford became more than a daydream I couldn't say. Perhaps because I wanted so desperately to do so that I didn't dare think about it.

Why Oxford? For regional and romantic reasons. The former practical, the latter frivolous. We had left Liverpool in 1935 to live at Broadway in Worcestershire, a village at the foot of the Cotswolds, hardly thirty miles from the university. By 1936 my favourite poem was Arnold's *Scholar-Gipsy*; by 1937 my favourite novel Compton Mackenzie's *Sinister Street*. From earliest childhood I had backed Oxford (in the twenties a consistent loser) for the Boat Race. In 1938 I and some of the seniors had been taken for a tour of the Morris-Cowley motor car factory at Oxford. On the way back, the headmaster stopped his car briefly in the High Street and showed us the cloistered quadrangle of Magdalen. I was hooked: thenceforward it was Oxford or nothing. So it came about that I grew up under the romantic High Anglican umbrella of Charles Williams and C. S. Lewis instead of the nonconformist puritan brolly of Professor and Mrs Leavis; a mistake, as I see now . . .

By 1937 I began seriously preparing for an attempt at Oxford. What Latin I ever learnt at P.T.S. had been forgotten. So I was farmed out for private tuition to one of the masters at Northampton Grammar School. Mr Peach not only taught me enough Latin in eighteen months to win the necessary 'credit' marking, but even induced enthusiasm for the language. Perhaps his two achievements go together. Another Grammar School master took me for French, in which I did less well, but well enough for matriculation purposes. Ever since I have had great respect for the quality of the education provided by grammar schools; but it must be remembered I was getting private tuition, that is to say the undivided attention of my teachers.

In 1939 I passed the Oxford Senior Local, winning credits in almost everything except arithmetic (I failed to get a single answer right). As a sort of insurance I also took Responsions, as the university entrance-examination of Oxford is called, and just managed to scrape by with the Latin unseen. All that remained was to find a college that would take me.

Before I took the Oxford Senior Local examination my mother went back to South Africa to rejoin my father. It was decided that I should accompany her, see my father, then return to school under my own steam. I was seventeen and had been at the deaf school for nearly three years.

The voyage back (again on the *Llanstephan Castle*) shook me severely. We were going by the West Coast intermediate route, calling at Ascension and St Helena. To this I had been looking forward. Yet the first week on board ship I found purgatorial. My trouble was a panic apprehension of people. When not with my mother I loitered from deck to deck, alone and wretchedly pretending not to be alone; incapable of nerving myself to make acquaintances, ultraselfconscious and at loss. Partly I felt alien among the hearing, just as I had felt, when first I arrived at Northampton, alien among the deaf. For three years I had been segregated, more or less, from the ordinary world; as hospital patients become institutionalized, so had I.

At Northampton, apart from the headmaster, his family and staff, we were fairly completely insulated from other hearing people. We met and spoke with almost none except when shopping on Saturday mornings. True, we played cricket and football matches against the local schools, but except on the field we made no contact with our opponents. In the holidays we were (or at least I was) more or less cocooned in a small circle of family and close friends.

It is not good for the deaf, especially at the impressionable age, to be always together: though where education is concerned it is difficult to see how this can be entirely avoided. It is hard for the deaf to resist the temptation to segregate themselves. Because the deaf find it simpler and easier to mix with the deaf than with the hearing their bias is to become a community within the community, consciously or unconsciously isolating themselves from the rest of the world. This is particularly the case with deaf children and adolescents. Deaf children, especially deaf-born children, cannot help behaving differently from hearing children. Yet this different behaviour is in part contagious. If deaf children are herded together it must inevitably accentuate those idiosyncrasies and mannerisms created by the condition of being deaf. Having no other models the children naturally imitate one another. This intensifies little peculiarities of speech and demeanour, which in turn helps the segregation process.

No one talks to a deaf person in exactly the same way as to a hearing person. At the very least he will speak a fraction slower, a touch more carefully; often he will exaggerate lip movements, expressions of the face, use gestures and signs where otherwise he would not. Inevitably, then, deaf children (deaf adults come to that) do not talk to one another in the way they talk to the hearing. Knowing the short cuts and tricks of visual communication they develop a different idiom in dealing with one another: which may become, as with us at Northampton, an argot, a tribal language. So that I sometimes think nothing is worse for the deaf than the company of the deaf. Too easily do we erect among ourselves our cosy house of dumb-crambo and retire into the security of a common disability.

The weather of the two worlds, of the deaf and the hearing, is different: in passing from one to the other you have to become acclimatized. The deaf do not, because they cannot, deal in the nuances – particularly the verbal nuances – of personal relationships. Their dealings are direct – may appear outrageously direct; their handshakes are ungloved. They have a naïveté, and also a plain honesty of intent, that often makes the polite wrappings-up of ordinary people seem, by contrast, hypocritical.

Moving from the deaf into the hearing world, I missed the freedom and ease that comes from being the same as everyone else. Because of my good luck, because I had become deaf fairly late in childhood, because I had the habit of reading, and because I had those invaluable three years at a hearing school where, if I did not learn much that was academically useful, my antennae were at least kept in contact with 'normal' patterns of life and behaviour, I found it easier than some of the others to integrate with the everyday world when I left school. From the day I entered the deaf school I had begun to live a schizoid life, to develop two simultaneous personalities. This happens, of course, to anyone who goes to a boarding-school, but not I believe to quite the same exaggerated extent. In my case there was the persona whose orientation was to the ordinary hearing world, and the persona I assumed in order to live with my deaf friends at school, to talk their language and conform with their outlook. This persona was as valid as the first. Had I gone on living with the deaf after I left school I think it might have become permanent. I do not know. When I went up to Oxford I resorted to private magic. I dropped the Christian name 'John' by which I was known at school and by my family. It was a symbolic exorcism of my deaf persona.

Seven

To live effectively is to live with adequate information.
NORBERT WEINER, *The Human Use of Human Beings*

EVEN today it is with effort that I bring myself to speak to a stranger. At sixteen my timidity was exquisite. Much may have been due to adolescent self-distrust but the main culprit was a feeling of differentiation, a sudden consciousness that I was deaf. This awareness now afflicted me like an unexpected sciatica. I had not felt like that as a child. But adolescence brings blackheads and social sensitivity, the one to exacerbate the other.

Once aboard the *Llanstephan Castle* I found myself faced with the choice of retiring behind deafness or participating in life, if only in the life of the ship. Sooner or later I had to begin to meet and talk to people; the sooner the better, the later the harder. It was a choice, I could see, that would determine the future.

But for the first time I became really cognizant of deafness, of being different. 'Being different' – a crucifixion in adolescence.

To myself I could make excuses. 'If I weren't deaf, what fun I'd be having.' 'It's not my fault, it's because I can't hear.' And so forth. The most insidious of temptations, this everlasting enticement to blame all troubles on the handicap. Luckily no perspicacity is needed to realize that once you get started on that tack, it's all up. I began to see that if I made deafness the scapegoat it meant a life of self-delusion, of hiding moral failure behind the physical defect.

Thus the voyage to Africa played an important if uncovenanted part in my education. What better practice-ground for mixing with a variety of people than the tourist class of a long-distance passenger-boat? There can be few other places where one is thrown into continuous, haphazard and inescapable social contact with strangers for weeks at a stretch.

I passed the first few days aboard ship in an excruciation of shyness and envy. Around me I could see people enjoying themselves, making friends; a freedom I coveted. I might have stuck to that gregarious soul, my mother, and through her met people; but that policy, I felt, would prove in the long run self defeating if I wished to be independent. It seemed necessary to learn to find my own friends by my own devices.

Now this shyness was not wholly due to adolescence or the sudden consciousness of deafness. And this consciousness of deafness was not a sensitivity about being handicapped; I had lived too long with it for that. My deafness did, and still does, often make me feel at a disadvantage; but that is quite a different thing from feeling inferior. What made me suddenly conscious of deafness, rather than sensitive about it, was the awful incertitude in which I found myself – not knowing what was going on. How can you break into a group of people, join them, introduce yourself, if you have no notion what they may be talking about? Specifically there was the realization that I had no idea how to strike up an acquaintance. How does one break the ice – what does one actually *say* to a complete stranger? Having started, what then? I was at a loss because I had no way of finding out except by trial and ignominious error. Deafness prevented me from overhearing how it was done. I had no idea whatever of the form, what the conventions might be, how to recognize, interpret, much less supply the nuances of the opening verbal gambit. Uncertainties of this kind, such gaps of common knowledge and experience, constitute one of the major irks of deafness. It is not hearing that one misses but overhearing.

I got round the problem by involving myself with a set of middle-aged bridge-players. With them, I guessed, bridge would be the focus of conversation; I did not guess wrong. These people – they can be found in the smoking-room of every liner – were fanatical addicts. In need of a fourth to make a table they would have roped in King Kong or the sea-serpent. They, and it was now we, played bridge solidly eight hours a day: morning, afternoon, and evening. I was chained to their baize cloth much as Colonel Copeman had chained me to his backgammon-board. This endless card-playing soon became a drag. But it gave me social experience of a sort, and with experience, confidence. I needed confidence.

From the bridge-players I graduated to younger, less hardworking society. On board there was a blonde, one of those blindingly alluring creatures that are too seldom met with in this vale of tears. She may have been nineteen. Every male on the passenger-list was at her feet and under her thumb. Except me – I hadn't the courage to come within six yards of her or even approach the periphery of the court with which she was surrounded. I kept my distance, which may have piqued the girl into resolving that my scalp was going to dangle from her belt with the others. Or perhaps she was simply good-hearted. Whichever it may have been I am still grateful. In mid-voyage, as the boat approached the equator, I noticed that whenever I caught her eye, or she caught mine, she smiled – a smile to sear a regiment. My reaction was to duck behind a ventilator or dive down a companionway. It never crossed my thought that I myself might be the target. So one day she had to take direct measures; crooked a finger; I was summoned. Like a mesmerized rabbit I obeyed; became thereafter slave and incubus. Wherever she went I shambled behind, exuding devotion like an overgrown dog. Callously I abandoned my bridge-playing friends to King Kong or the sea-serpent; became one of her entourage and began to enjoy myself immensely.

By the time we disembarked at Table Bay I had broken my heart; when it mended, I found I had been de-institutionalized. My 'I am different' attitude, and fear of people, had almost gone. But I knew it could easily recur. I made up my mind to keep in practice and never again allow myself to revert to the shell of deafness; to talk to people, especially strangers, at every opportunity.

The South African vacation lasted three months. Christmas found me with my father and mother in an old Army bell-tent near Knysna; at least my mother slept in the tent, my father and I *à la belle étoile*. (This did not prevent our Christmas turkey, that hung from a tree adjacent, from being stolen in the night. All Christmas day we fished for our dinner; but caught nothing, so had to drive to the nearest town for a square meal.) I was taken to see fantastical accretions of stalagmite and stalactite in the labyrinthine Cango Caves; to the ostrich farms under Zwartberg and to the snake park at Port Elizabeth. Then home to Johannesburg, that year celebrating its fiftieth anniversary with a grandiose fair, of which I remember little except a miserable family of Bushmen from the Kalahari who were kept on show in a compound as if they were animals. After the fair was over I spent weeks there with my friend Billy – by then an electrician's apprentice – helping to dismantle booths and show-buildings. Johannesburg appeared full of Germans; the swastika flew beside the union flag on the town hall. Before I left for England a few weeks were spent with cousins at Broken Hill, in what was then North Rhodesia and now is Zambia. Inconceivable that within thirty years it would be an independent state· for the whites seemed more dominant there than in South Africa itself. Perhaps I was misled, as the white races often are, by the mere politeness and good manners of the inhabitants. If I walked along a country lane they would kneel and solemnly clap hands in greeting. And one day, strolling down a road on the outskirts of Broken Hill, I saw a native approach on a bicycle. He stopped, dismounted wheeled the machine past remounted and rode off. Apparently it was disrespectful for a native to remain in the saddle in the presence of the master race Yet it was in this then remote corner of the sometime empire, at a tobacco-farm in the middle of the bush that first I came upon 'modern poetry' in the shape of a copy of Harold Munro s anthology of twentieth-century verse. The poem that caught my imagination was *Tristan da Cunha* by Roy Campbell, of whom I had never heard. Among other Rhodesian wonders I took in the grave of Cecil Rhodes, a megalomaniacally reticent bronze slab forever alien on a dome of bald granite, surrounded by great boulders like giant marbles; Victoria Falls with its pall of cloud, the condensed spray sent up by its mile of fallen water; its delicate bridge clasping the gorge, and incongruous palatial hotel which boasted (so they told me) the northernmost water-closet on that side of the equator. Then I sailed back to England on the *Balmoral Castle*. My mother remained with my father in South Africa. This voyage I made entirely on my own. For the first time since becoming deaf I was completely independent and responsible for myself.

In England I now lived, when not at school, at Broadway in Worcestershire. With my aunt and an Anglo-Indian cousin I lodged at the house of one of my mother s friends, an old colleague from Guy's Hospital. The village stood at the foot of the northern scarp of the Cotswolds, on the main road from Worcester to London. To the west lay the Vale of Evesham and the isolated whale's back of Bredon Hill, behind which on a clear day you could see the blue line of the Malverns. The south and east were dominated by the low northern edge of Cotswold hovering above the midland plain like a comber about to break. On the highest point of the scarp, directly over the village, stood Broadway Tower: a round battlemented folly looking like the letter l in lower-case. For ten years this village remained more or less my home.

The rail journey between Broadway and Northampton was complicated. It was on a certain section of this line that, six times a year, I religiously fulfilled my vow to practise talking to chance companions. The scene was the local connexion between Leamington and Blisworth Junction. This train consisted of two or three corridorless coaches drawn by an antique steam-engine whose design – particularly the long smokestack like an early Victorian tall hat – approached that of Stephenson's Rocket more nearly than anything I have ever seen actually moving on a railway. Her beat was twice a day from Blisworth to Leamington and back, for which reason she was known to her regulars as Wandering Lizzie. She never broke down but made each trip an act of faith. On starting, gouts of steam puffed from her engine's every nook and cranny, tube and joint: volleys of smoke billowed from her teetering funnel. Steam and smoke obliterated the platforms; till in the end she began to heave creakingly off, like an old lady hoisting herself out of an armchair to fetch a kettle. Once away she became surprisingly skittish. She would rattle along at a disreputable pace, clattering over level crossings, wheezing long woolly skeins of thick white smoke that went lolloping over fields and paddocks as, gathering speed, she clanged and jingled, snorting smuts and fiery sparks and thoroughly enjoying herself. An hour later she would subside panting at the terminus; absolutely pooped.

On this train I kept my hand in, and guarded against a return of social paralysis, by forcing myself to buttonhole anybody unfortunate enough to find himself or herself in my compartment. No doubt on occasion hands strayed in the direction of the communication-cord, but nobody actually pulled it – perhaps fearful of the effect on the bundle of old pistons and leaky pipes gambolling in front of us. In fact I was never rebuffed, and found most of my victims surprisingly patient and sympathetic.

Less sympathetic, though not unreasonably so, were the authorities of the university which I was now seeking to enter. In the thirties it was hard to get a place even as a commoner at any of the Oxford colleges; though not nearly as difficult as it seems to be nowadays. I do not know very much about the negotiations that went on between my headmaster and the principals of the various colleges. But the fact that I was deaf, if not absolutely a liability, did not exactly help. The Rector of Lincoln pointed out, with reason, that I would indubitably be run over in the street before I had been at Oxford a week. However, the authorities at Oriel seemed willing to take a chance. I believe it was to the then Vice-Provost, M. N. Tod, that I owed my eventual acceptance by Oriel College. At least he allowed me to sit for an examination for one of three vacant places at Oriel. In 1939 there were some sixty candidates. Mercifully nobody told me that there were only three places to be competed for (a fact I did not learn until long after I had left Oxford). The examination, which took place in the hall of Oriel, I supposed to be more or less a formality. Even so I was nervous enough. About the examination I remember nothing except that at one point I had to write an essay of some sort; what the subject can have been, not the remotest notion remains with me.

Like most of her alumni I associate Oxford with melancholy, probably because the opening term begins in autumn. Mist rises from the river, leaves are umber and falling, college passage-walls glisten with damp, the days shorten, it rains. Approaching Oxford the train halts for two minutes' rumination by the cemetery. The first notable building on which the eye alights after leaving the station turns out to be the city jail. All the preliminary impressions contrive to be lowering.

Mine may have been more than usually so because I arrived at the beginning of the first term of wartime. Half the colleges had been requisitioned either partly or entirely by an embattled bureaucracy. One of these was Oriel. With other Oriel freshmen I boarded out at Hertford College, where I was assigned a dark and dingy pair of rooms on the ground floor of its New Buildings. The romantic vision of a mullioned study window dreaming over a medieval quadrangle collapsed with a sigh. Hertford's New Buildings had been designed and built less than ten years before, but remained, however, authentically medieval in plumbing and what are called conveniences. None of the rooms had any of the former; as for the latter, these were represented by a corrugated iron shed in a back alley.

Despite requisitioning and blackout, the afterglow of *l'entre deux guerres* lingered. There was no rationing; lush four-course breakfasts were served in hall, with lunches and dinners of proportionate magnificence. Most of the second-year and many of the third-year undergraduates had come up, either to finish their courses or to mark time till they were summoned by one or other of the armed services. A number were exempt from conscription – those taking medicine, science, or divinity for example. (They could, if they wished, volunteer; and after the fall of France many did.) For the first two terms of wartime the university remained more or less its peacetime self.

Going up to Oxford was like emigrating from Tristan da Cunha. I was totally ignorant of the manners and mores of the males of my own generation. As for the other sex, I found myself incapable of the most perfunctory social relationships with any unattached member of it under the age of thirty-five. Introduced to one, I would shake hands, say nothing whatsoever, slowly but remarkably assume a sunset tinge, and stand there thinking furiously, until such time as the girl's nerve broke and she fled, leaving me undisputed master of the field. It was two years since my voyage to Africa, and though I had practised buttonholing strangers to keep my social hand in, most of the confidence acquired on the *Llanstephan Castle* had dispersed. Oxford was a world so strange that I would in any case have been terrified. I knew nobody there of course. What I was really frightened of was committing any kind of solecism, slipping up on some arcane point of etiquette. I imagined myself surrounded by Etonians, viscounts, God knows what, every man jack on the alert for the least breach of the social code. I could feel their eyes burning holes in the back of my best blue serge suit. As when, dining in hall one evening, I recollected that I was wearing a pair of brown shoes with it, whereupon the food turned to ashes in my mouth. After dessert I slunk off, convinced that one and all had seen, noted, and condemned the sartorial faux pas. This was the kind of suffering I created for myself.

Niaiseries I can hardly bear to recall: such as the day when I wanted a needle to sew on a button. Having no idea where to buy one I wandered into the most palatial draper in Cornmarket. The manager, beaming, approached me in his frockcoat, washing his hands in the air:

'What can I do for you, sir?'

'I want to buy a needle.'

Worse was my interview with my 'moral tutor' at Oriel. His name I forget – now I come to think of it we only met on the one occasion. The function or duty of a 'moral tutor' was to look after the well-being and well-behaving of his undergraduate protégés. I had not been up for more than a day or two before mine requested me to pay him a visit. The interview was a fiasco, entirely through my fault. Unable to lipread the man, I would not admit it but pretended to understand where I didn't. Within fifteen minutes we tangled ourselves in an inextricable, not to say surrealistic, mesh of cross-purposes. Half an hour later, exhausted, we parted with the usual polite expressions of farewell – perhaps the only lucid exchange of the encounter. Why didn't I ask him to write what he had to say? Nerves mostly: and because I had begun by bluffing, letting him think I was au fait with what he was talking about in the hope of picking up the clue sooner or later. Too soon it was too late; we reached the point of no return, when it would have been unforgivable to confess I hadn't understood a syllable and had been wasting everybody's time. On this occasion the situation was complicated by a hallucination that afflicted me after the first few minutes. I convinced myself that my tutor must be talking about one of the staff of P.T.S. who had been at Oriel (and so, I supposed, known to my 'moral tutor'). Once you get a hallucination of this sort almost everything you 'read' on the other person's lips appears to confirm its authenticity. The mind makes the eye see what the mind expects. I believe my 'moral tutor' came to the conclusion (who can blame him) that I was off my chump.

As for the academic aspect of my life at Oxford: long before going up I had decided to read English. Or rather, had decided (like many who take the Honours School of English Language and Literature) that it was the only subject I had a chance of getting a degree in. Later I thought this decision was a mistake, that I should have taken history instead and so gained a solider background for the Eng. Lit. that I would in any case have read. Had I the equipment I would have liked to take Modern Languages. But my French was just about good enough for the School Certificate, no more; and there was the point that I couldn't pronounce a word of it. (When I try to speak French, for some reason the only people who understand me are Italians.)

The thing that bothered me before I came up to Oxford was, what to do about lectures? Like so many problems in life this one resolved itself. For my first term I attended all the lectures I was supposed to, following the shoal of English School freshmen from hall to hall, from lecture room to lecture room. My solution was the obvious one of asking a neighbour if I might copy his notes as he made them. For me there was no question of being able to lipread the lecturers. But, apart from the drawback of having to depend on the note-taking efficiency of whomever I chose to sit next to, I found the whole business too cumbersome and time-wasting to persevere with. Much the same information, it seemed to me, I could get out of the Bodleian in half the time. I agreed with T. L. Peacock – 'Those who do not understand the subject will not understand the lecture, and those who do will learn nothing from it' – though in holding that opinion I was probably making necessity a virtue. In my last year, before the examinations, I borrowed and studied three years' lecture notes, but without much profit. What I did learn at Oxford, which is I suppose the valuable lesson of a university, was how to instruct myself, how to set about collecting the knowledge and material I needed. This is the best aspect of the tutorial system as I experienced it.

Two tutors were assigned to me – one for Anglo-Saxon, one for Eng. Lit. John Bryson of Balliol was my Anglo-Saxon tutor; an Irishman, and as much interested in the contemporary arts as in the Old English poetry through whose allusive intricacies it was his task to navigate unenthusiastic undergraduates. He was not noted for his punctuality, or rather, the organization of his time – when taking my weekly essay to his rooms, which were in the Victorian Gothic part of Balliol at the top of a spiral stone staircase, very narrow, and chill, and steep, I would likely as not find myself stumbling over recumbent bodies still keeping vigil for their tutorials. One of them had inscribed on the wall a pencilled modification of Milton:

> Avenge O Lord thy slaughtered saints, whose bones
> Lie scattered on this Alpine staircase cold . . .

Yet Bryson illumined for me the gnarled enamelling of Old English poetry, in particular *Beowulf* – which, long after, I was to translate into modern English in an attempt to get away from the Butcher-and-Langery, and self-conscious poetrifaction, of other versions. For many years this translation was to earn me an income, modest but substantial enough to form the basis of a living while I went on learning to write verse. My other tutor was a clergyman – a retiring, modest, obstinately conscientious character. He said little, but what little he said had acumen; words that lodged in the mind, even if – as usually I did – one disagreed with them at the time. One morning I burst in on him –

it was the summer of 1940 – with a mind occupied not with Augustan poetry but with newest bad news:

'Paris has fallen.'

'Indeed, Mr Wright. Kindly let me hear your essay on Pope and Warburton.'

His doggedness was reflected in an incident that occurred at his church (he was vicar of a small parish near Oxford). A new stove had been installed, and on the first Sunday after it had been put in he took the service as usual. Not long after he had mounted the pulpit to preach the sermon one of the congregation fainted and had to be carried out. He paid no attention to the interruption, even when, a little later, another worshipper also fainted and was similarly dealt with. One after another his flock began to diminish, but he carried on till finally no one was left but himself and two or three of the congregation who had been busy conveying the insensible bodies of the rest into the open and laying them out in the churchyard. There they soon revived, for they had been only temporarily knocked out by carbon dioxide fumes from the new stove, which, being heavier than air, affected only the seated congregation and had not reached the pulpit. When I read this story – for the papers got hold of it – I had to salute the inflexible tenacity I knew so well.

The tutorial system consisted, so far as I was concerned, in my writing an essay once a week for each of my tutors on some theme or thesis they proposed. They would suggest a reading-list (one was expected to improve on it). Thus I learned to hunt through libraries, to get up a subject, to quarry for material or (after all, I was taking Eng. Lit.) opinions. I had to read the resulting essay aloud to my tutor and subsequently digest or endure his comment. The tutor would then mark the essay with some arcane Greek lettering followed by a mathematical symbol. Here I may confess that I did not then understand what these meant and never asked. Some inane sensitivity about my unorthodox or at any rate non-public-school education held me back from confessing ignorance; so to this day I have no idea whether my tutors thought my essays competent or the reverse.

What I missed through not being able to follow lectures I can't and won't presume to judge. But the tutorial system as it existed at Oxford in my time might have been tailored for my particular disability. It was in effect individual tuition. Where that is lacking any deaf student must be at a disadvantage; but wherever it exists he has a fair chance. Of my academic education there is little more to say. I took my finals in the summer of 1942 and came off with a second-class honours degree: I didn't expect or deserve a first.

But I did not then regard, nor do I now, the academic side as having been the real and valuable education a university should offer; it was part but part only of what I hoped to draw from a place like Oxford. The rest and best of it must, even then I realized, come from the people to be found there, from contemporaries. It is not, finally, from one's elders that one learns. In this sense my education continued long after I left Oxford.

For the first couple of terms my main preoccupation lay in mustering the nerve to approach people, to talk to them, to find out, in fact, how life is lived. For, sheltered at the deaf school and by the family group I lived with at Broadway, I knew nothing of it and knew that I knew nothing. How different life is from the depiction afforded by novels – even the great ones – then my prime source of information. Years later John Wain was to appal me by remarking that he read novels in order to find out the kind of world he lived in.

If I got into casual conversation with somebody, say a neighbour at dinner in hall, I would pester him to come round to my room for tea some evening. My aim was to get a party of seven or eight together so that conversation might be general and none need feel embarrassed. Behind this screen I would tackle each guest individually with what I presumed to be acceptable chat. Some of it must have been pretty weird. At that time I had the notion, God knows where I got it from, that undergraduates addressed one another as 'Sir' in the course of ordinary conversation. And I remember my perplexity when somebody (a divinity student, come to think) used the word 'cunt', and neither he nor anybody else would tell me what it meant.* I even joined the college boat club and learned to row. Not that I had any particular enthusiasm for this on the whole pointless form of exercise; but it served as a plank for making acquaintances. And I

---

* Like so many deaf, I missed all schoolboy bawdy and was well into my teens before I understood 'the facts of life'. I don't think it made much difference one way or another: though at Oxford I was for a while a diligent researcher into what was then the last stronghold of oral literature, the blue story and the blue limerick, to me novel art forms

needed every plank I could get, for I still had to screw myself up before passing a remark to anyone. In my first term days often went by without my exchanging a word with a soul – until boredom overcame timidity.

Rowing was my choice partly because I loathed football and most other games; partly because I thought it might please my father, who had rowed for a Thames boat club; and partly because rowing seemed the romantically appropriate pastime at Oxford. It chanced that at that time Oriel was the crack rowing college, having gone over to the Fairbairn or Cambridge style a year or two earlier. The last two Boat Races had been won by Oxford eights dominated by Oriel men, thus breaking an interminable succession of Cambridge wins. I was taught to row Fairbairn by one of these Old Blues; and almost caught the infection. Certainly I caught influenza.

This was the result of a dip in the river in the February of 1940, the hardest winter since 1928. One freezing foggy afternoon I was rowing no. 5 in the second eight on a practice outing. Chunks of ice, miniature icebergs, could be seen floating down the Isis, whose banks were shrouded with fog as well as snow. There were times when the coxswain, Ken Pinnock, could barely see a length in front; and at one such moment he ran the boat's nose into the bank. Of this I was hardly aware; the bump might have been another block of ice, a theory that seemed confirmed by a particularly large one sweeping past my seat, followed by a few bits of wood which looked as if they had once belonged to a boat. They had; and what's more, they had belonged to our boat – part of the bows had been carried away. Next moment we were up to our waists in water. We abandoned ship; all but Ken Pinnock, who couldn't swim. He and the half-submerged boat, oars splayed every which way like the legs of a drowning beetle, began drifting rapidly downstream. Those of us who had reached the bank plunged in again to bring the vessel and its shivering pilot safe to shore. In the course of this rescue I was nearly killed: by the University Trial Eight, no less. It came shooting under Iffley Bridge and was upon us before anybody realized; or rather upon me, for the long sharp bows, like the horn of a swordfish, came shearing through the water at a good twenty m.p.h. straight at my head. I had no time to feel frightened; just enough to think; 'This is it', when all eight oars simultaneously hit and held the water – an imperious foaming splash like an alighting swan – and brought the boat to a dead stop within a foot of where I was floundering. Dramatic stuff.

Among the rowing men I got to know the public-school types. I found myself admiring them immensely – the 1939–40 crop, at any rate. Nearly all were waiting to join the air force, and nearly all, it seemed, were to be killed in the Battle of Britain or shortly after. They were, I suppose, bloods; I was an oddball. The Oxford climate changes quickly: a few years before such misfits as myself would have been ignored, or if not ignored, subject to horseplay (debagging, room-wrecking) from 'hearties' of their type – or so I am led to believe by the memoirs of some of my thirties predecessors at the university. These, on the contrary, behaved with the greatest kindness. They never seemed to mind me hanging around but would even ask me to their rooms for drinks and parties, a thing that meant much at that time. One has been put off by the Hillary cult – most of my rowing acquaintances were contemporaries, and some may have been friends, of Richard Hillary – but this particular generation had a magnanimity of spirit which I never again encountered. They lived with zest, as if they felt in some way set apart, which in fact they were.

Very gradually I began to find my friends and feet. The friends I made were generally offbeats like myself. For some reason most of them were biochemists. One was Gerhard Schmidt, a refugee from Berlin. This was the man who used to play Bach's Italian Concerto for me on the piano. He had come to England as a schoolboy, knowing no word of the language. Because of this he may have understood my communications problem better than most. English he had mastered in a few months by a simple and Teutonic expedient; he learned a dictionary by heart. 'The first week, everything I said began with A.' From his conversation, which was mordantly funny, and from that of his biochemist friends, I learned all that I ever knew of scientific method. Through Gerhard I was to have the experience of sitting out one of the first air-raids on London in a cellar full of Germans – it gave piquancy to the self-congratulatory eulogies of British phlegm under fire that appeared in the papers next morning. He was shipped off to a concentration-camp in Australia after the fall of France, but returned some eighteen months later when that particular panic had subsided. This Australian concentration camp seems to have been a university in miniature: for the young intellectual élite of the German-Jewish refugees to Britain all found themselves dumped there. Many became Gerhard's friends, and after their return, mine too; among them the polylingual, immensely read Georg Rapp, now a publisher. Rapp introduced me to two very odd fish indeed, both older men and, in their different ways, both poets. E. W. H. Meyerstein I met once only, but never forgot. He had a lumbering unhappy body, a knotted spirit crucified by a literary acumen that deserted him in the face of his own verse. The other was the most unremittingly unlucky human being I ever knew; gentle, wizened, as if shrivelled by the Nazi holocaust that consumed his family in Czechoslovakia: the anthropologist Franz Steiner, then writing his classic and caustic examination of taboo. Characteristically Steiner was to lose the manuscript of this book in a railway-train, together with all the notes – representing years of reading – on which it had been based. His poems, unlike poor Meyerstein's, deservedly received recognition when they were published in Germany some years after Steiner's death. Another odd man out I came to know well was an engineer, a Rhodes scholar from Malta, the son of a sea-cook (literally: his father had been one in the Royal Navy). He was at Hertford, and like myself rather a fish out of water. We got into the way of talking far into the night over pot after pot of tea – the same tealeaves wetted again and again, for the sake of economy and rationing – sessions wherein he would speak of the poetry of Leopardi (he almost got me to learn Italian) and expound what he meant to do on his return to Malta: raze the slums of Valletta, reorganize its Labour Party, and generally get things moving in the right (or properly speaking, left) direction. The last time I saw Dom Mintoff all this had come to pass and he was the then prime minister of Malta.

Not a few were made uneasy by my deafness, however. In those days I was made uneasy by it myself, which didn't help. A minor ordeal for any naturally shy person is confrontation with a deaf man. Often I mistook such shyness for a brush-off, or worse. But I was given insight into one kind of reaction that someone like myself can provoke, when it occurred to me to ask one of my closest friends at Oxford what he had felt when first we met. His reply was:

'Resentment.'

'What do you mean?'

'I resented somebody like you coming into my life.'

That was a disconcerting and valuable remark. I realized that I should often have to manage this natural if unflattering initial response from people. Yet, looking back on my life, it seems to me that when I was young deafness acted as a kind of filter. It constituted an unintended but effective litmus-test of anyone I met. As I have noted, one runs the risk of looking slightly ridiculous or at least of appearing at a disadvantage when dealing with the deaf. Thus the self-important, the self-regarders, and those careerists whose interest in people is in their use or status, did not much trouble themselves with me, so I did not much trouble myself with them.* In this way I gravitated towards offbeat types – unless of course I am deceiving myself and it was my own inbuilt offbeatness, rather than deafness, which was responsible.

The war got worse; rationing came in; the friends I made in my first year were called up, or shipped off to Australia; some got killed. I had an agonizing love affair, which was followed by an agonizing love affair. The turnover of undergraduates, who now arrived for no more than a couple of terms before being called up, became so rapid that I found myself promoted Captain of Boats. In this unlikely eminence I acquitted myself with inadvertent success. Called to attend a meeting of Captains of Boats, I misunderstood what had been decided and trained my wretched crews to row the full course (a mile or more) for Torpids. In reality the race was over the half-course, which fact I did not discover till the day it was rowed. As a consequence all the Oriel boats won by at least six lengths, which pleased the crews so much they forgot to curse me for the extra and unnecessary labour I had inflicted on them during training. I did less and less work as I came into contact with more and more people. In my last year at Oxford I moved into digs at 52 High Street.

This proved my introduction to the literary set at Oxford,

* I am not going to carry this autobiographic sketch beyond my time at Oxford, but may note here that later on, when again entering a wholly new society, the London literary scene of the forties (albeit I came in by the back door, the Soho pubs), I could not help distinguishing between those who took the trouble to speak to me and those who had no time to waste on an obscure deaf youth nobody had heard of. The behaviour of genuine artists (nearly always they were poets) was consistently magnanimous.

which I had more or less avoided, perhaps because poetry was my sacred or at any rate secret preoccupation. For at the same time that I moved in the room under mine was taken by Sidney Keyes, who was then, in succession to Keith Douglas, the reigning Grand Cham of Oxford poets. He had edited for Routledge a decorously produced anthology called *Eight Oxford Poets* in which appeared the verse of Keith Douglas, Drummond Allison, John Heath-Stubbs, and Keyes himself. No. 52 High Street naturally became their headquarters. An inauspicious address as it turned out; nearly all the Oxford poets who took digs there in the forties were allotted early and violent deaths. It might have been taken as an omen when, in the first month that Keyes and I lived at No. 52, the third lodger, a Magdalen undergraduate, threw himself into the Cherwell one night and drowned. Barely a year after he left Oxford Keyes was killed at the tail-end of the Tunisian campaign, while his friend Drummond Allison (who inherited my room) died a few months later during the Italian landings. Neither was older than twenty-two. Some time after Allison's death his room was taken by William Bell, a poet whose potentiality may have been greater than that of either. Bell died at twenty-four, killed while climbing the Matterhorn. This last fatality was too much for Mrs Taylor, our landlady; appalled at the rate of mortality, she thereafter refused to take on any more undergraduate poets.

Keyes's poetry – at the time he was scarcely nineteen – was extraordinarily assured and polished; it hypnotized his contemporaries. Sooner or later everyone, including me, found himself writing Keyesian poems whose chief characteristic was a kind of romanticism one associates with the paintings of Fuseli. Dialogues in verse between two stock figures, of whom one was inevitably Death and the other invariably a Lady, accompanied by an imagery of skulls and grails and swords and similar furniture, were the thing. To be fair, the poetry of Keyes's immediate circle was least characterized by props of this kind. This circle included Michael Meyer, John Heath-Stubbs, and Drummond Allison. Allison's poems, scribbled in the most horrible handwriting I have ever seen, were if anything anti-romantic. They have survived on the page where the mannered elegance of Keyes has faded. But Allison was the least literary of the group – in jargon, he was an extrovert; a rackety *enfant terrible* with tow-coloured hair. I would see him disappearing into coffee-shops or emerging from pubs with fabulous beauties from the Slade.* Then there was Michael Meyer, blond and plump, who was later to emigrate to Sweden and translate the plays of Ibsen into what remains the best acting version in English. The other member of the group was John Heath-Stubbs, whom I now met for the first time, though like everyone else at Oxford I knew him well by sight. No one who ever set eyes upon it could forget that long, lean, lanky, almost disarticulated figure flitting along the pavements of the High like a heron or a flamingo about to take wing; which would suddenly stop dead, petrified in every limb, then warily permit its head to revolve, scanning the horizon from left to right while the remainder of its body stayed rigid; thereupon, with the abruptness of an electric hare at a greyhound track, to scoot off again at forty miles an hour for the next thirty yards, when the process repeated itself. Heath-Stubbs was even then nearly blind, and even then an immense storehouse of information on matters vegetable, animal, and mineral, while his incomparable collection of theological data concerning the various Christian (Roman, Coptic, Orthodox, and of course Anglican) faiths with each and every of their attendant heresies, was already forming. Then if one wanted to listen to an unrivalled orchestration of superb and weirdly reverberating substantives one had only to get him going on the classification of birds – to ask him, say, for an anatomical description of the skeleton of a great bearded tit.

I never got to know Keyes very intimately, and doubt if anybody did. He was a solitary, the very opposite of Drummond Allison. It seemed to me that for Keyes poetry and art were a means of fencing himself off from life, rather than an instrument for exploring it. I usually saw him late at night, when I would drop in on my way to bed, and we would have a cup of cocoa in either his room or mine. As I never learned to lipread him our conversations took place on paper. Some scraps have survived, but they are not of much interest. It was Keyes, now I think of it, who introduced me to the poetry of Dylan Thomas (not too enthusiastically) and of Vernon Watkins, to whose first book he had given an encomium in Cherwell. Apart from Yeats and Hardy, my own reading of what used to be called 'modern' poetry had

* The Slade School of Art, transferred from London to Oxford for the duration. In the war years we were lucky to have endless supplies of beautiful girls, art students from the evacuated Slade and similar institutions, who had nothing to do with the university, but let a little air into the place.

begun at Oxford – for at Northampton the work of Ezra Pound, Joyce, or even Eliot (to say nothing of Auden, Spender and Co.) never came my way. In those days contemporary poetry enjoyed nothing like the publicity and general accessibility it has now. My first year at Oxford I spent in soaking up Eliot, Joyce, and Pound in that order. Keyes and Heath-Stubbs awed me with the extent of their reading; especially Heath-Stubbs, to whom I must ascribe a large part of my early literary education – but that took place in London, at the university of Soho.*

Just as Cobber Kain (anyone remember him?) was publicized as the first air ace of the Second World War, Sidney Keyes, as its first young poet of any note to be killed, became its Rupert Brooke. After his death in 1943 a posthumous collection of Keyes's poetry was awarded the Hawthornden Prize. He was compared with Donne and Rimbaud; but today, despite a recent biography by John Guenther, his poetry is practically forgotten. Yet he had the luck to have enjoyed, as it were, his posthumous reputation while still alive. For at Oxford his name was legendary. In those days a factitious awe attached itself to the name of a poet, the more so if the owner of the title were young and awaiting call-up. Our generation, after all, had come to Oxford to find still freshly engraven on the various college war memorials the names of the dead of just two decades before. The image of Wilfred Owen and Isaac Rosenberg, if not of the less intellectually respectworthy Rupert Brooke, was at the back of everyone's mind. (And the newspapers kept asking: 'Where are the war poets?' with indignant glances in the direction of America, whither one or two of the better-known literati were supposed to have scarpered.) In those days the popular conception of a poet, before it was superseded by the beer-and-bedlam Dylan legend, was firmly fixed to the Keats-Shelley image. It became Keyes's

* The pubs in Rathbone Place (technically not in Soho at all). During the war and late forties Soho was a meeting-place for writers, painters, musicians, and all sorts and conditions of people from every quarter of the globe. It was the lineal successor of Montparnasse of the twenties, some of whose survivors (e.g. Nina Hamnett) had transferred to Soho. One could meet literally anybody there, the King of Poland, a Cambridge Senior Wrangler, or the fighting forces of half Europe. The decline began in 1950 when 'Soho' moved south of Oxford Street to wash against the north side of Shaftesbury Avenue; thereafter espresso-bars, pop-musicians and purple-heart cafés took over. But it was in Soho, rather than Oxford, that my friendship with Heath-Stubbs began.

destiny to fulfil the public requirements for a war poet; and through his early death he fitted the bill so neatly that it is only with conscious effort that I now recall he did not, in fact, carry about with him the affects of a doomed poet but of an all-round man-of-letters.

It was about the time I met Keyes, though not because of it, that I decided poetry was to be my vocation. I never had any idea, throughout boyhood, what I was going to do for a career. Deafness, as good an excuse as any, eliminated most jobs. Inability to answer the telephone crossed out the idea of office or business employment. I had no interest in and less aptitude for most of the trades and professions in which deafness would be least a liability: farming, market-gardening, architecture, cabinet-making, forestry, printing, engineering, chemistry, and so on, to name a few that my fellow-pupils at Northampton went in for. I could not even serve behind a counter; but at a pinch would be able to work as a dishwasher. These reflections ought to have worried me more than they did. But my targets had always been limited ones – first to matriculate, next to get into a university, next to get a degree. As to what would happen after I got the degree, I never really thought about that. Having decided, rightly or wrongly, that the writing of verse was to be the main preoccupation of my life made the question of a 'career' of less interest or importance. Somehow or other, I supposed, I would make or get enough money to live on. Looking back I am appalled at this optimism and its justification. In life if you want a thing badly enough you are liable in the end to be given it, suitably wrapped by the ironic gods. So be careful what you want.

It was not through the Keyes circle that I began to find my way to the people under whose aegis I finally grew up. Just before I met Keyes I got to know Cyril Frankel, who had come up to Oriel in the summer of 1940. My friendship with him developed in much the same way as that with Dom Mintoff. Frankel had not been at Oxford a week before he set about founding the Oxford University Ballet Club. For this he organized a series of dances by two members of the Ballet Rambert: Sally Gilmour, then its prima ballerina, who had made her name in Andrée Howard's *Lady into Fox*; and Walter Gore, today one of the best and the most neglected of English choreographers. After seeing their first performance (Gore's *Bartlemas Dances*) I was made captive; and thenceforward, for the next seven years, a balletomane. Cyril Frankel invited me to hitch-hike with him at week-ends to whatever town or city the Ballet Rambert happened to be visiting. Frankel used to wear his o.t.c. cadet's uniform, against all military law, to facilitate the hitch-hiking. This made it a nervous business; we had to keep a look out for the redcaps. Once in a cul-de-sac near Cardiff, catastrophe stared us in the face, in the shape of a platoon of marching soldiers aimed directly at us. As the o.t.c. uniform would have got Frankel into serious trouble had it been spotted, he was about to freeze behind a dustbin (the only available cover) when, with precise last-minute timing, as in a Mack Sennet film, the squad halted, right-about-turned, and marched off in the reverse direction, leaving Frankel pale and shaking against his garbage-can.

At this time Walter Gore was beginning his career as a choreographer. He found the O.U. Ballet Club useful for try-outs – among them the idea of ballet danced to the spoken word. This was well before Robert Helpmann of the Sadler's Wells used the same idea for his ballet of Milton's *Comus*. At Oxford I saw the first performances of Gore's *Porphyria's Lover* and *Confessional*, danced to the words of the poems by Browning. Walter Gore was a quiet man. We often found ourselves sitting next to each other at the innumerable parties Cyril used to give. From that companionable silence – we inclined to watch rather than talk – sprang a friendship. It was developed by a long correspondence that grew up between us – Gore liked to spill his ideas on paper in my direction. Then one day he asked me to write a poem for a ballet. My first professional commission. Eventually I turned out *Minster Lovell*, a shockingly romantic piece full of Keyesian imagery and based on the legend of the Mistletoe Bough. The scenery and costumes for the ballet were to be designed by Honor Frost, then living at Oxford to help Benno Elkan with the casting of the pair of bronze candelabra now in Westminster Abbey. Nothing came of the scheme* but through it I came to know Honor Frost.

Even then she was a remarkable woman: designer, painter, sculptor, and typographer; besides being as beautiful as only

* At least not immediately. The ballet was eventually created, but given a new title – *Ginevra*. It was first performed at Amsterdam, then at Lisbon in 1966, the poem having been translated into Portuguese for the occasion. Hardly what had been envisaged in 1941; but perhaps it goes to show that no work is entirely wasted.

intelligent women can be (or is it vice versa?). Later – having become one of the first to take up skin-diving – she was to pioneer the techniques of underwater archaeology, to excavate (if that be the word) shipwrecked Greek and Roman galleys off the coast of Provence, and sunken harbours off the Turkish littoral; her book, *Under the Mediterranean*, is the first and most authoritative work on the subject. It was to Honor Frost that I owed three introductions, each of which, one way or another, proved decisive. The first was to David Gascoyne, who took a room in Wellington Square for a few weeks in the summer of 1941. I had not then read a line of his verse (indeed had never heard of his name) but in him I recognized the authority of the real thing. Gascoyne was intensely nervous, tall as a pylon, beautiful as a derelict angel escaped from the illuminated margin of an Anglo-Saxon psalter. He talked (or rather wrote in his elaborately rococo script, for I could not lip-read him) of Valéry and Kierkegaard. From him I learned that poets do not have careers. The second introduction was to Tambimuttu. At that time he was operating from a ratty old basement cellar in Chelsea, where he lived on visions and unsold copies of *Poetry London*. He was a Ceylonese; and his function that of a catalytic agent. In the disrupted years of the war he ran one of the only two 'little magazines' entirely devoted to verse. But the influence of his magazine, good or bad, was nothing; Tambi's service lay in his role as a kind of peripatetic rendezvous, a one-man Institute of Contemporary Arts through whom, at a time of scattering and regimentation, poets and painters met one another. He kept the lines of communication open. You could call him the Lady Ottoline of the Second World War, not least for his eccentricity and enthusiasm; not to mention the eccentricity of his enthusiasms. Soho, sleazy and rumbustious, was the Garsington where he dispensed Dutch hospitality. The third and last introduction was to the Coffee-an', an unbelievably bohemian underground café off Soho, where the stage was set for the annihilation of a protracted adolescence.

Eight

We speak with our vocal organs,
but we converse with our entire bodies.

DAVID ABERCROMBIE, *Paralanguage*

HERE I call a halt to autobiography. My life after I left Oxford
had less and less to do with deafness and deafness less and less
to do with my life. Many do not escape so completely, certainly
not as easily. For the deaf-born, to break through the silent cur-
tain and 'pass for white' among the hearing is a much tougher
proposition. On this account I have to thank my luck that deafness came upon me after I had learned language in the normal
way, by ear; that I retain some subliminal awareness of the tone
and natural rhythms of speech.

. It has also been my luck to be, or at least to want to be, a poet.
A *sine qua non* of the vocation is obsession with language and
words. As Auden put it, 'Good poets like bad puns'. I cannot tell
whether deafness has damaged my poetry, but I know that
poetry has damaged my deafness. Because words and language are
its medium they are my predilection – or perhaps it's the other
way about – for which reason I lose no chance of picking up their
living use. Catchphrases, nonce-words, nonce-jokes, current
idioms, vogue expressions, new coinings, regional usages, even
dialect – I am a compulsive snapper-up of all unconsidered vernacular trifles wherever they are to be found. Often I find them
in the course of ordinary conversation but, knowing how much
casual talk I miss, I am continually on the look out and seek my
quarry where I can – letters, newspapers, comics, novels, plays,
strip cartoons, pop songs, advertising copy, notice-boards, hoard-
ings, labels, instructions on the packet, lavatory graffiti – anything available in writing or print. This kind of exercise, whether
or not I have been able to turn it to good account as a poet (a
point not here under debate), has done as much as anything to
keep my conversation colloquial or at least unstilted, and myself
au fait with the verbal environment.

Everyone who writes verse thinks of himself as a poet. I did at school; but it was not till I was twenty that I began to understand that the vocation, like the name, may be conferred but not assumed. However this is not an aspect of my life that belongs to the subject-matter of this book. Yet I should perhaps attempt to explain how, though not why, one as deaf as myself manages to write verse. There is, as I am fond of recalling, the precedent of Ronsard and du Bellay. I can only say that I do not think deafness comes into it very much. I hear a noise in my head – a music? a rhythm? – and have to find words that fit, or recreate, or express, that rhythm or music. As George Barker once described this initial process:

'It's like listening to a long-distance telephone call on a bad line.'

People wonder how Beethoven composed his music after becoming deaf; I don't; for, as I should know, it is not necessary to be able to hear in order to hear.* The inner ear exists as much as the inner eye; and what Wordsworth calls 'the mind's Internal echo of the imperfect sound' as well as the 'eye-music' he spoke of, the transmutation of movement into apparent sound, by which the visible appears audible. Then I have a feeling for rhythm – like many of the deaf, I am a quite good dancer.† And there is that inexplicable quality of poetry, which hasn't, I think, been sufficiently investigated: its ability to survive in different pronunciations. It is known that the pronunciation of English has changed over the centuries; if we had a record of Pope reading *The Rape of the Lock* he would sound queer, and Shakespeare speaking one of his sonnets queerer yet, while Chaucer might be unintelligible. But the sound-effects of their verse do not seem impaired by modern pronunciation, or at least not fatally. There is dispute about the true pronunciation of dead languages like Latin and ancient Greek, yet the auditory qualities of the verse of Homer and Virgil are praised by those who cannot be sure how it

* In any case Beethoven would have been able to *feel* the vibration of most notes in the scale, except the very high ones.

† I discovered this accidentally as a young man – accidentally, for I had taken it for granted you could not dance if you could not hear the music. A girl persuaded me to try, and I found that I could very easily and quickly pick up from my partner the rhythm of whatever tune was playing. With a bad or uncertain partner I can make do by watching the movement of other dancers from the corner of my eye. The better my partner dances, the better I perform – and, of course, vice versa.

was spoken. For myself, without a notion of the proper pronunciation of French, I obtain great pleasure from the auditory quality of the poetry of Racine; yet the sounds that I read from a line like

> *Mais tout dort, et l'armée, et les vents, et Neptune*

can only bear the most distant and distorted relation to the sounds indicated by Racine's notation. I have no explanation to offer of why this should be so.

I am not claiming that deafness makes *no* difference, or even that I rely wholly on what I call my inner ear, as far as the fashioning of my own verse is concerned. There are words in my vocabulary which I have never heard or seen pronounced, so that I cannot be certain on which syllable the stress falls. I have had to get round this trap by writing much of my verse in syllabics (i.e. using the count of syllables as a frame, rather than a count of stresses). There is a failing which I condemn when I come across it in the work of some contemporary poets, yet inevitably find difficult to avoid or get rid of in my own: a tendency to fall into a 'literary' style – in other words, to use the idiom of written rather than spoken language. Finally, as in my own verse I dislike using full rhymes except on rare occasions (they always sound too heavy), I find I have evolved a peculiar, or perhaps idiosyncratic system of near-rhyme, or vowel rhyme, similar in effect. It was a long time before I discovered the principle behind these near-rhymes – why they 'worked'. They were, I realized, a kind of eye-rhyming – not rhymes of words with similar spelling but different pronunciation (like 'though' and 'through') but homophones, or *lipreader's* rhymes. The rhyme is in the lip-movements. I do not use this kind of rhyming systematically (poetry abhors a system) but here is an example: a stanza rhyming *abab* –

> No I am not speaking of professional bohemians
> Of those who mine for status in the stratas of culture;
> I mean those who are not in the service of a competence
> But of an extraneous vision, of an idea.

One way to forget one is deaf (or blind, or a dwarf, or whatever) is to have to concentrate on making others forget it. Most of my life, apart from adolescence, I have not often been consciously aware of deafness. Sometimes this obliviousness rubs off on other people – witness an involuntary compliment I have worn like a medal since the day it was handed me by a casual pub acquaintance. He was a man I used to drink with from time to time in Chelsea. One evening he offered me a free ticket for a piano recital in the Wigmore Hall. Then he saw my expression.

'Oh my God. I quite forgot. I'm most terribly sorry.'

He went on apologizing, convinced that he'd dropped a brick; it was a gold brick.

After leaving my deaf school laziness prevented me 'keeping up my speech' by taking lessons or even by practising the elocution exercises we used to be given. Yet the surprising thing is that it did not deteriorate but actually improved. Of this I have objective evidence. During my last year or so at school I noticed that people who did not know me (shopkeepers, bus-conductors) had trouble understanding what I said. After I had been at Oxford for a few terms this no longer happened. Now I am not implying that our speech was neglected at school or that elocution exercises are useless. My better articulation was due, I believe, to the fact that I now lived in a hearing milieu. The best speech exercise is speech itself. I no longer had the temptation or opportunity to slip into lazier habits – for example, the voiceless enunciation I find myself adopting when talking to a deaf friend. So long as I get the lip movements right he will not know or care whether I produce the correct noises. But when talking with the hearing there are no short cuts; one must speak properly, or else. Besides which one is unconsciously absorbing natural speech rhythms to the benefit of one's own.

Except for a few school friends that I occasionally ran into, and one or two people I met like the deaf-born A. R. Thomson, R.A. ('I don't know whether I'm coming or going,' as he used to say), I have lived almost exclusively among the hearing since leaving Northampton. At one time, before I found my feet at Oxford, I was wary of slipping back into the easy but limiting world-within-world of deaf companionship. There was, in my time, another deaf undergraduate at Oxford: neither of us made any attempt to meet, though we knew of each other's existence. This man had become deaf at seventeen and was taking a science degree; I heard of him through my biochemist friends. I think we both instinctively felt that our kind of battle was best fought alone at that stage of our lives. Years afterwards we corresponded – by this time my companion in silence had become a Fellow of the Royal Society. Towards the end of my third year at Oxford an Oriel friend who had already gone down wrote me up anonymously in the *Volta Review*, the leading American magazine for the deaf. I knew nothing of the article until one afternoon I found a white-haired, furiously energetic old gentleman waiting for me in my digs at 52 High Street. I was completely foxed when he began by attempting to communicate by means of the finger-alphabet – this was in fact the first time I ever saw it used by an expert. We found each other mutually incomprehensible, and talked, if that is the word, at crosspurposes. Then for a week afterwards clergymen, mission workers, and God knows what came knocking at my door offering help and pamphlets, invitations to join deaf-and-dumb clubs and one thing and another. The old gentleman's name was Selwyn Oxley, a famous philanthropic worker among the deaf, as long afterwards I learnt; but at that time I had never heard of him. He was as much outside my experience as I appeared to be outside his. Despite the *Volta Review* article which had prompted him to seek me out, he seemed to assume I had little or no command of language, or at least of spoken language. Perhaps he was too used to the often inarticulate deaf among whom he worked; a world with which I had no contact.

I did not take up the invitation to join the deaf-and-dumb club; I felt it was not my scene. Later, in London, I heard of the Spurs Club from some old school friends who had become members. Founded in 1934, it is perhaps the best and best-known of clubs for the deaf. Yet it is not a deaf club, but a hard-of-hearing club: a distinction which has nothing to do with the amount of hearing the members possess, but everything to do with their modes of communication. Deaf clubs are for those who use the finger-alphabet; hard-of-hearing clubs for those who speak and lipread. In the latter sign language and finger-spelling are banned. Some of them, really intended only for people who have become deaf late in life, will blackball anybody who like myself has been educated at a deaf school, no matter what his attainments. The ostensible reason is the fear that such a person might introduce 'signing', but I should think that it is really because the recently deafened and lifelong-deaf have usually little in common. Different communications, different lives. The gulf between the speaking and the signing deaf, and again between the lifelong and the lately deafened, can be deep and wide.

Deafness has effects over and behind the obvious ones, yet I do not think it alters character. Rather it intensifies those elements already present – making the pessimistic more pessimistic,

the selfish more selfish, the sanguine more sanguine. I speak of
the deaf from childhood rather than of those who lose hearing
in middle age. Two friends of mine, both at Northampton with
me, seem to have been born with a natural goodness and gaiety
of disposition which their deafness appears to leaven rather than
diminish, somehow protecting the native innocence of their
characters from corruption and deterioration despite the ordinary disappointments and matters of grief that life and fortune
bring. On the other hand the bitterest man I know is a deaf man.
His bitterness has no good reason, his life having been successful and fortunate except for deafness; but then I do not except
deafness.

About the relation between the hearing and the deaf I know
nothing at first hand, for it is as a deaf man that I meet the deaf.
But I once observed an intimate aspect of it – the relation of
hearing children to deaf parents. It was a family I came to know
well: both parents deaf-born, the children perfectly normal. Nothing impressed or moved me more than the reciprocal guardian-
ship existing between the children and the parents, the
interdependence of responsibility on each side. When I first met
them the eldest boy was about eight or nine – there were two
younger children. The father was an architect. The boy, I noticed,
made it his business to look after both his parents as far as the
missing sense was concerned – he dealt with the telephone and so
forth. This was less remarkable than the tact and unassertiveness
with which he managed to be indispensable; yet there was no
diminution of ordinary high spirits or of the exhilaration natural
to his age. Most very young children, as I know from experience,
are good and quick at dealing with the deaf as soon as they understand the situation. So I was curious to know how early the boy
had discovered his parents' deafness.

'Oh, he found out we were deaf when he was a little baby,
before he could speak,' replied the mother.

'But how could you tell he knew?'

'It was easy to tell. When he was a few months old, he stopped
crying. You see, he found out it was no use crying if he wanted
us; he used to beat me, or the pillow, with his arm instead. He
knew we were deaf, he never cried again.'

Deafness can be a stimulus – at least I have found it so. Always
it has dangled in front of me, from my teens into middle age,

the experience of ordinary life as a supreme or almost supreme desideratum. Ordinariness, the extraordinary aspiration of cripples! Because not to be attained, or at least not without effort the commonplace and banal become invested with glamour. Thus there are experiences I owe to deafness in so far that had I not been deaf I might not have gone out of my way for them. Cut off from part of the experience life offers by the obstruction of one sense, you are made greedy for the remainder. My maxim has been: Who am I to say no? not the best, but not the worst of guide-lines.

Among oblique effects of deafness: extreme gullibility, at least so far as concerns the spoken word. Anything that is *said* to me I take as gospel: the spoken word carries the mystique and prestige attributed to print by the half-educated. Probably for the same reason: the effort and exiguous feeling of achievement that the deciphering of the written and the spoken involves for each.

Among minor annoyances: inability to follow or to join in group-discussions, the to-and-fro of argument. The full attention must focus on a single interlocutor; thus all conversations, even in crowded rooms, are virtually tête-à-tête. Then again, not being able to turn the eyes away from the speaker, even to glance about to take in one's surroundings, to sense the mood of the company by noting the way people are standing, moving, behaving. One has to adopt certain tactics that seem rude if clumsily done. Arriving at a party, I try to avoid speaking to anyone for the first minute or two in order to absorb as much visual information of this sort as possible; for once engaged in conversation I can't. At a dinner-party or a luncheon, where one's position is going to be fixed for the next hour or two, I have to manoeuvre like the vainest of spinsters for a seat with my back to the light: for I must see people's faces.

Moments when most aware of deafness: when I cannot follow what is *not* addressed to me. Not being able to overhear, rather than not being able to hear, is the real turn of the screw. Being overheard is a related problem. For I have no judgement of how far the voice can carry, or of what noises may mask it. In crowds, or where people are about, the instinct is to lower the voice particularly when what I have to say is not meant for the general ear. Conversely my impulse is to raise it in empty places or where no one is around. So I have an involuntary and maddening tendency to whisper at parties but shout in churches. I do speak up at parties when I remember or am reminded – to be disgraced, now and then, by those inexplicable silences which sometimes fall on gatherings of people; always, it would appear, in the middle of one of my more scatological remarks.

Another ungetridofable delusion: that out of sight=out of ear-shot. Because I equate sight with sound, the moment someone passes out of the field of vision my reflex is to assume I am inaudible. If I am talking to someone and he turns a corner or disappears behind a door or screen, I involuntarily stop speaking. Even though I know he can hear me, my subconscious won't believe it. Walking with people at night, in the dark, I fall silent; so strong is the reasonless conviction that hearing depends on seeing. This phenomenon a friend once dramatically made explicit. I was inflicting on him some monologue; while I spoke, he abruptly covered his mouth with his hand, whereupon I automatically shut up. The moment my view of his face was obscured it seemed as if the lines of communication had been cut. I don't know which of us felt the more surprised.

One or two friends are in the habit of addressing me without giving their words voice, partly because they find I lipread better and partly because they like the mystification it occasions, as when I am trapped into making, seemingly apropos of nothing whatever, some surrealist pronouncement for the edification or astonishment of bystanders. There is a pub between Penzance and St Ives whose landlord used to believe that he had three regulars of whom only one could utter a word, the other two being deaf and dumb. My two companions were, of course, sound in tongue and ear . . .

Yet I have never reached a high standard of lipreading. Some attain a proficiency that appears miraculous, especially to one like myself who knows what is involved. A friend of mine (now a leading architect in South Africa; born deaf, he had a far harder row to hoe than I) seems able to read almost anyone, even at a first meeting; and what's more, from angles so extravagant that in effect he is reading, not the mouth, but movements of the jaw. Another man lipreads three languages – French, English, and Russian. Not long ago I met Dr Pierre Gorman, a deaf-born Australian with a Cambridge doctorate, at a meeting of audiologists at Edinburgh University. Dr Gorman astonished me by sitting through the entire meeting (it lasted all day) and following the various speakers apparently without effort, despite the highly technical language some of them employed. Even if I had had his skill I doubt if I could have stood the strain of so many hours' concentrated lipreading. When I made some admiring remark about this feat, Dr Gorman seemed surprised.

'You ought to be able to do the same. Relaxation is the secret.'

Dr Gorman, I am sure, is right. When in any state of tension, nervousness or over-anxiety, I have the greatest difficulty in following anybody, including my nearest and dearest. On the other hand a drink is a great help to lipreading, obviously because alcohol relaxes tension. This is not an illusion, for when well away I have performed prodigies in this field that are beyond me in normal circumstances. It's one reason why I spend so much time in pubs.

I began these chapters of autobiography by observing that up to the age of seven I had been exceptionally lucky; concluding them, I find I must amend the remark. After the age of seven I was even luckier. This is not a question of looking on the bright side. I was lucky in my parents, in my schooling, even in my deafness.

For handicaps of this kind bring with them a consolation, albeit of a left-handed sort. Consolation is not the right word; it is more in the nature of a quid pro quo. The handicapped are less at the mercy of vague unhappinesses that afflict so many, especially those without aim in life, whose consequent boredom promotes what used to be called spleen. The disabled have been given a built-in, ready-packed objective which is always present: a definite impediment to get the better of. Like the prospect of hanging, it concentrates the faculties wonderfully.

After forty years of living with it, I can only write as one attuned to, not protesting against, the state of deafness. For me what is interesting about it is less the nature of the condition than the point of view it obtains. Like an eccentrically-sited camera taking angle-shots that distort but may often reveal otherwise masked lineaments of truth, the deaf person watches from the unexpected and unguarded quarter. It is to this aspect of deafness, rather than its miseries and consolations – which are not so very different from the miseries and consolations of other infirmities – I would draw attention.

For the notion that the loss of one sense is offset by an augmentation of the others is a mistaken one, at least in my experience. Were it true, then after forty years' deafness I ought to be exceptionally observant, but I am not, though sometimes appearing so. What has happened is that I do not notice more but notice differently. I observe objects and people as such in the vague and general way common to most persons. I could give no more than the feeblest description of the street I have lived in for twenty years, while my memory for faces is plebeian. What I do notice, and notice acutely because I have to, because for me it makes up almost the whole of the data necessary for the interpretation and diagnosis of events, is movement where objects are concerned; and in the case of animals and human beings, stance, expression, walk, and gesture. As Freud once put it, 'If a man's lips are sealed he chatters with his fingertips.' For example, as somebody waiting impatiently for a friend to finish a telephone conversation with another knows when it is about to end by the words said and the intonation of the voice, so does a deaf man – like a person queueing outside a glass-panelled call-box – judge the moment when the good-byes are being said or the intention formed to replace the receiver. He notices a shift of the hand cradling the instrument, a change of stance, the head drawing a fraction of a millimetre from the earphone, a slight shuffling of the feet, and that alteration of expression which signals a decision taken. Cut off from auditory clues he learns to read the faintest visual evidence. The deaf man can, if he knows his friend intimately, make a good guess at the identity of the caller at the other end of the wire. He will do this by noting his friend's expression, or the tempo of animation in his countenance; the posture of his body (relaxed or tensed); and what his hands are doing. For people tend to turn different facets of their personalities to their various acquaintances. This orientation of personality is expressed not only by the adoption of a slightly altered tone of voice and style of conversation, but by infinitesimal adjustments of the lineaments and carriage. The latter are not generally observed, since most people are naturally attending to other sources for the same information. But the deaf person notes them because they are the only signals he can receive and interpret. Since few, apart from professional actors, realize just how much stance and carriage of the body reveal of mood and emotion, even when the expression on the face is assumed or disguised, it can happen that by the paradox of his disability the deaf person is often in the position of an eavesdropper listening to what he is not intended to hear.

In all this there is nothing extraordinary. It is simply the attainment of the same objective by a different and more round-about process, like getting a cork out of a bottle with a knife when the proper tool is not to be had. A man without a corkscrew soon becomes handy at using a substitute. The deaf person does not have a keener eye but has had to cultivate a special attention to ascertain the answers to questions posed by inaudible phenomena. Outside the range of his necessary curiosity he is likely to be as unobservant as anybody else and as hard put to it as the next man to notice whether or no his wife is wearing a new hat.

As regards the techniques and pitfalls of deafmanship: always the most exacting challenge is making acquaintance with a stranger. The chance that X may turn out to be a bore or otherwise undesirable is one that besets all men; but what bothers the deaf buttonholer is the risk that X may turn out to be difficult or perhaps impossible to understand. Almost certainly X will be hard to follow to begin with; inevitably so for moderate, not to say mediocre, lipreaders like myself. People's mouths differ in shape and character, as do their ways of speaking. Regional or national accents like the American/Irish flat 'a' constitute another hazard. Thus it generally takes time to pick up the idiosyncrasies of the lip movements of a new acquaintance. If one is lucky X may turn out to have a deaf friend or relation. In this case X will be a more or less 'trained' speaker, for those who have to do with the deaf usually acquire a knack of clear enunciation. If X is one of these I can tell in a moment. Or he may be an actor. Actors are dead easy for lipreaders because elocution is part of their trade. After all you can't make yourself heard in the gallery unless you open your mouth a bit. But with most people it's a toss-up whether they're going to be no more than reasonably difficult to follow, or hopeless cases who grinch language between gritted teeth. If the latter, what to do? Produce paper and pencil with a charming smile – though generally I find myself producing the charming smile, having lost or forgotten the paper and pencil.

One ought at once to admit to deafness. One seldom does as one ought. My own strategy allows X to run on, in the often justified hope that I'll begin to pick up the thread. Meanwhile I can read his expression, catch his tone from his face. Unless I have to I will not let the deaf cat out of the bag. This is partly vanity, partly a curiosity to see how long I can get away with it; and to some extent because acknowledgement of deafness must momentarily unbalance the relationship so far established.

'I'm afraid I'm deaf.'

Whereupon X, if he has never before come across a deaf as distinct from a hard-of-hearing person, will raise his voice, perhaps shout. Here is my cue to explain that all he need do is speak with care, and not too fast. Let me make a clean breast of my lack of manners: more often than not I ruthlessly fail to take the cue. For the louder people speak, the more they use their mouths; teeth-gritters will even unclench their jaws. The more they shout, the better for the lipreader. I am now able to follow X, whose enunciation has been made visible as well as over-audible. But things may cancel out – for example if X begins to lean closer and closer to my ear to further the work. At all costs I must keep my line of vision to his face; so I step back. If this is a badly managed encounter we may now begin to perform a kind of slow tango. Here is X advancing on my ear, myself retreating step for step, eyes fixed on my partner's face . . .

Aside from such farces, the point at which I acknowledge deafness is the moment of crisis. It cannot help but embarrass X. All he can say is:

'I'm sorry.'

Though why he should be is never clear. There may be a built-in animal reaction that makes us resent, just a little, disability in another. Wolves turn upon a wounded member of the pack. *Homo sapiens* does not go that far, but the subconscious response, however minimal, however overlaid with inhibitions and social or ethical training, however instantly disguised as pity, is of the same order. May I remark here that I take no offence at this split-second of unconscious illwill. Why should I, when myself I experience it when meeting a hunchback or a blind man? It exists; the task is to dispel the transient awkwardness that it generates. One way is to talk about deafness. Besides helping to dissipate embarrassment, the information may be useful to X. And once he realizes that deafness is of no great moment to me it ceases to worry him.

As I have repeatedly observed I am not a particularly good lipreader – or it may be that from the lipreading point of view I find myself at the receiving end of somewhat difficult conversations, by virtue or vice of the company I keep. The easiest kind of talk to follow – if the least rewarding – is the tattle-tea-party sort. Built up as it is like a Meccano toy out of standardized interchangeable sections or clichés, it is only necessary to 'read' a word here and there to guess the rest of the sentence.* At any rate, of the people I meet, I find about half mostly unintelligible, because they either don't enunciate or have a distorting accent, or talk too fast, or simply because it takes time to get the hang of the way they speak. Where familiar friends are concerned the picture is of course different (though there are some I still cannot lipread, after twenty years) and indeed I find it easy to follow their talk even when they are speaking fast. This occasionally leads to an unexpected kind of social embarrassment at parties or in pub conversations where a stranger joins in. Such are the operations of the human ego that if what is said by the stranger is not understood with equal facility – for though he may realize one's deafness, he probably won't be aware of the factors contributing to the difference between lipreading a familiar acquaintance and somebody new – he often feels affronted. For the good reason that nothing is less pardonable to the vanity than that somebody should appear to refuse one's own communications while accepting another's.

Lipreading is not simply a question of interpreting movements of the mouth alone. The intonation of the voice must be read as well. Someone for example says,

'You bastard.'

This conveys nothing unless the accompanying emotive qualification is obtained. What is meant by the expletive phrase may be admiration, gratitude, chagrin, or disgust, entirely depending on the tone used by the speaker. The most obvious visual clue to the emotion qualifying the spoken word is the expression of the eyes. So in lipreading one actually focuses one's attention on a speaker's eyes rather than his mouth, reading below the line as it were the verbal enunciation of his mood. Communication involves more than language, it is the sum of what is being felt as well as said. This is so much the case that I find myself completely unable to lipread anyone whose eyes I cannot see – somebody wearing very black sunglasses for example. In the same way the eyes of blind men often throw one off. They are expressionless because they cannot react. The divining of people's moods and

---

* On the other hand the toughest lipreading assignment is to try to follow a quotation from an unfamiliar poem. In poetry the words have, or should have, the quality of being both right and intellectually surprising, so the dice are loaded against guesswork.

intentions from their eyes is so much easier (since it makes less intellectual demand) than the reading of their actual words that it is possible (I do it frequently, when tired or bored) to sustain a conversation without really knowing what is being said. A few noncommittal interjections graded in tone to match the temper of the other person's expression are all that is needed to maintain the illusion that one is following his conversation. If it is a funny story he is telling the task is even easier. The mounting tempo, the crinkle of risible muscles as the nub of the joke approaches, are easily read warnings to be on hand to laugh at the pay-off. The danger is that one may be asked a direct question when one has no idea what the conversation is about. The best gambit is to reply 'Well ...'

Give it a long pause and nine times out of ten the other will be happy to start answering the question himself.

For the truth is that people want to communicate more than they desire communication. It may seem a paradox, but the deaf person – so far from being liable to be left out – is often in a strong position psychologically, like a mountain surrounded by Mahomets. Though this is only true of those who have dominated, not merely accepted, the disability. Every disability offers the same alternative: either it dominates you or you dominate it. This truism is demonstrated every day, not necessarily on the heroic scale of Wing-Commander Bader or the late Helen Keller.* A corollary is the fact that once a disability has been dominated it ceases, truly, to be a disability but becomes an asset, a weapon, like the blind eye of Nelson at Copenhagen.

Deafness is of course very much a nuisance and its disadvantages are severe. The blind and deaf Helen Keller said that she found deafness worse than blindness. I wouldn't agree, though in combination the deafness must obviously weigh more heavily. Among the minor but none the less oppressive afflictions that deafness entails I would note the continual drain of energy. When not alone one has to be on the *qui vive* all the time; that and the effort of lipreading are nervously exhausting. Then there are the irritations, like missing a train because one has not heard the Tannoy announce that it will leave from a different platform or at

* Not to mention Arthur MacMorrough Kavanagh (1831–89) who, born without arms or legs, learned to ride, fish, shoot, write and draw. He was an M.P. for fourteen years and travelled widely in Egypt, India, and the Middle East.

a different time. And the telephone poses its problems apart from the disadvantage (if it is a disadvantage) that no one can ring you up. You can get people to ring up for you, but this expedient is an invasion of one's independence; it is embarrassing to have to ask the same person to perform the chore too often. Then you may want to ring X, but cannot ask Y to do it for you because Y has fallen out with X; while Z is out of the question because you may not wish your business with X to be known by Z. Harder to bear as one grows older is the boredom one must often endure for polite or social reasons, for example when visiting someone's house and the hosts and other guests wish to listen to music or a radio programme. In such cases there is nothing to be done but sit it out as inconspicuously as possible. Besides being a matter of courtesy it is important not to embarrass people with one's disability when this sort of situation arises, or you find yourself a drag on people's enjoyment. It is one thing to use your handicap as a weapon and another to lay it on other people's shoulders as a burden.

Apart from such vexations and impediments the life is not essentially different from other people's: full of worry and passion, pleasure and boredom, all of it one's own fault or contriving. It only annoys to have a special quality, 'courage', attributed (as it often is by people who like to patronize) to the fact that one has become adapted to the conditions of a peculiar existence: as if everyone did not have to have courage in order to be alive at all. There is a story about Sigmund Freud that bears on this. Somebody was telling him of the fate that had befallen one of his old friends, a Swedish professor I think it was. This professor was in the middle of writing a book when he had a stroke that left him paralysed, able only to move his eyes. However he went on with his work, dictating the book to a secretary by the laborious expedient of directing his glance from one letter to another of an alphabet painted on the wall opposite his bed. The man who told this story asked Freud,

'Don't you think that's a supreme example of courage?'

'Of course I don't,' said the psychologist 'What else could he have done?'

Second Part

By the Effigy of St Cecilia

Having peculiar reverence for this creature
Of the numinous imagination, I am come
To visit her church and stand before the altar
Where her image, hewn in pathetic stone,
Exhibits the handiwork of her executioner.

There are the axemarks. Outside, in the courtyard,
In shabby habit, an Italian nun
Came up and spoke: I had to answer, 'Sordo.'
She said she was a teacher of deaf children
And had experience of my disorder.

And I have had experience of her order,
Interpenetrating chords and marshalled sound;
Often I loved to listen to the organ's
Harmonious and concordant interpretation
Of what is due from us to the creation.

But it was taken from me in my childhood
And those graduated pipes turned into stone.
Now, having travelled a long way through silence,
Within the church in Trastevere I stand
A pilgrim to the patron saint of music

And am abashed by the presence of this nun
Beside the embodiment of that legendary
Virgin whose music and whose martyrdom
Is special to this place: by her reality.
She is a reminder of practical kindness,

The care it takes to draw speech from the dumb
Or pierce with sense the carapace of deafness;
And so, of the plain humility of the ethos
That constructed, also, this elaborate room
To pray for bread in; they are not contradictory.

Nine

THUS far my own personal experience of deafness. Had I been born a hundred years earlier – in 1820 instead of 1920 – my history must have been much less fortunate. At any rate there would have been no chance of a university education: little beside the most elementary teaching was then available for deaf children, and in 1820 the number of schools offering even this could almost have been counted on the fingers. For the beginning of secondary education for the deaf was still a matter of living memory when I left my Northampton school in 1939. And in 1942, when I took my degree at Oxford, I could claim a place among the half-dozen or so pupils from a deaf school ever to have graduated at an English university. Even the legendary Abraham Farrar, the first to achieve this, was still living. That is in itself a commentary on the recentness and difficulty of the higher education of the deaf.

Today, if not exactly commonplace, it is not out of the ordinary for the deaf-born, or those adventitiously deafened in childhood like myself, to attend universities. There are now two secondary schools for the deaf in Britain, besides one grammar school, the Mary Hare Grammar School for the Deaf at Newbury. It may not sound much, but compared with the situation barely a quarter of a century ago represents huge improvement. The list of public examination successes achieved *annually* by pupils at the Mary Hare Grammar School is half as long as the whole of the 'Roll of Honour' that used boastfully to hang in our classroom at Northampton. Yet this is far from a reflection on my old school, for that 'Roll of Honour' represented perhaps as much as eighty per cent of the public examination successes of deaf pupils in Great Britain between 1881, when Farrar matriculated and entered London University, and 1939, when I went up to Oxford.

In America a deaf-mute man gained a university degree for the first time at Harvard in 1902, followed a few years later by the triumph of the blind and deaf Helen Keller, who graduated *cum laude* from Radcliffe College in 1908. Today more than ten per cent of the students at Gallaudet College (since 1864 the only college for the deaf with a right to confer its own degrees) go on to graduate at ordinary colleges and universities, while a sizeable proportion of pupils of the many other U.S. deaf schools, like the famous Clarke School for the Deaf at Northampton, Massachusetts, do likewise.

Like no other class, the deaf depend on education for their integration into society. This is particularly the case with the deaf-born, who, it is seldom realized, are more helpless than the blind, being cut off from the beginning from the means of communication, even of communication with themselves. Who were the obscure pioneers who first tackled the intractable problem of providing the incommunicable and uncommunicating deaf with the means of breaking or reducing their isolation from society? Cardano, Bonet, Amman, Dalgarno, Pereira, Braidwood, de l'Épée, Heinicke, Gallaudet, Arnold, Alexander Graham Bell – barely half the rollcall of names in this little-known and neglected field of endeavour – yet perhaps only the last has even been heard of by most people. When in 1928 Miss Neville arrested the growing inarticulateness of my speech, and when in 1934 I entered the Northampton School for the Deaf, I benefited not only from my immediate teachers but from the work of their predecessors. These pioneers laid the foundations of the insights, techniques, and skills from which I profited, and which today are being modified and expanded in the light of technological advance. And it may be that the most objective way of illuminating the problems set by deafness, and the means by which they are combated, is to trace the history of the education of the deaf from its beginnings to the present day.

The school at which I was educated had its place in that history. The continuity intrigues me as I reflect on two visits, more than twenty years apart, that I paid to its successor, the Mary Hare Grammar School for the Deaf, in 1947 and in 1969. For eighty years the Northampton school had been the first and only establishment in Britain to send deaf pupils – albeit only a handful – to finish their education at universities. It had been founded in 1868 by the Rev. Thomas Arnold, one of the earliest pioneers of the higher education of the deaf. He had trained and been succeeded by his assistant, H. N. Dixon, who in turn had trained and been succeeded by Frederick Ince-Jones, my old headmaster.* But in 1944 the Northampton school had to close its doors owing to the illness and retirement of Ince-Jones, who for forty years had been an unremitting champion and practitioner of Arnold's aims and principles.

At the time, so far as higher education was concerned, the only real competitor of the Northampton school was Miss Mary Hare's Dene Hollow Oral School at Burgess Hill. That too came to an end in 1945, when Mary Hare died. Many of Ince-Jones's pupils had come to him from Mary Hare: a mild rivalry subsisted between them, though the Burgess Hill school was co-educational and run on very different lines. This remarkable woman had opened her school as long ago as 1883, first in London, then at Brighton, transferring it in 1916 to Burgess Hill, where she continued to run the school till she died – over sixty years of continuous teaching; an awesome record. Mary Hare left her estate as the foundation for the first national grammar school for the deaf in Britain. The proposition had been made more feasible by the 1944 Education Acts, whereby the duty of providing secondary education for all children in Great Britain was laid on the local authorities. ('There was nothing in the Acts,' as the writer of a recent survey of deaf education blandly remarks, 'to suggest that secondary education in some form should not be provided for hearing-handicapped pupils.'†) Thus the Mary Hare Grammar School for the Deaf first opened its doors in 1946 at Burgess Hill. It was not, and is not, controlled by any local education or county authority but by its own Board of Governors and Trustees, though the pupils' fees are paid – as the Education Acts lay down – by the local authorities in whose areas their parents live. None other than E. L. Mundin, who had been trained by Ince-Jones and had been his assistant for more than twenty years at the Northampton School for the Deaf, became its first headmaster.

A year after the new school opened I went to see my old teacher

* I regret, now, that I never met Abraham Farrar, the school's first pupil, as I might easily have done. Certainly I would have questioned him about the Rev. Thomas Arnold, and perhaps have been able to preserve some personal reminiscences. Ince-Jones sometimes talked about his predecessor, 'who really preferred botany to teaching deaf boys': he was a specialist in lichen and fungi. As a teacher of the deaf Dixon was eccentric in that he wore a beard, giving as a reason: 'If my boys can lipread me they can lipread anybody.'

† T. J. Watson, *The Education of Hearing-handicapped Children* (University of London Press, 1967).

at Burgess Hill. There were forty or so pupils – twice the number there had been at Northampton. Mr Mundin, full of plans to move the school to Arlington Manor near Newbury in Berkshire, had been enthusiastic about the possibilities and scope offered by its much larger premises and the great park of woodland and pasture in which it was set. I promised myself a visit when the move was accomplished to see what had been done.

But I never saw Mr Mundin again. Very soon after the school transferred to Arlington Manor in 1949, what would have been a valuable and brilliant career was abruptly foreclosed. One day Mundin went out into the park with a shotgun for rabbits; as he was negotiating some hedge or gate the gun went off and killed him. He was forty-five. Not for two decades did I pay my self-promised visit to the school. One January afternoon in 1969 I found myself being shown round it by the principal, Mr Askew, Mundin's successor and former colleague. In the panelled dining-room Mr Askew pointed out to me a link with Northampton and Arnold: a posthumous oil-painting of the first headmaster of the Mary Hare Grammar School. There were the neat features of my old teacher Edgar Mundin: recognizable, yet unlike.

The same might be said of the world of deaf paedeutics I was revisiting after so long an interval. A month earlier I had been asked to address a conference of the newly-formed British Society of Audiologists at Edinburgh University. This was a meeting attended by headmasters of deaf schools, audiologists, phoneticians, linguists, and physiologists. I may say that I was as much surprised as intimidated to find myself addressing so learned a gallery. (You may well wonder how I came to be there at all. As with most of the turning-points of my life after I left Oxford, I can trace the determinant to the years I spent in the pubs of Soho. I had been roped in to the conference through the agency of Professor David Abercrombie, the head of the Department of Phonetics at Edinburgh. (Had it not been for his brother, the late Ralph Abercrombie, whom I first knew at the Black Horse in Rathbone Place, the professor might never have heard of me.) As my function at the conference was to provide a subjective element to balance more objective studies of hearing and its disorders, I read an extract from the opening chapters of the present book – the descriptions of the experience of deafness and its onset. This was the first time I had ever undertaken to read in public. Quite frankly I did not think I would be capable of speaking for twenty consecutive minutes (the length of my paper) and still be articulating coherently at the end of it. But all efforts on my part to have my paper read by proxy were gently but inflexibly opposed by the organizer of the meeting. As it turned out soon after I began reading I warmed to the work, and – so they told me – ended by speaking more distinctly, than when I began. Probably I was helped by the interest, albeit professional, that I could sense being extended to me as I read. But that is by the way.

This conference gave me the opportunity to meet for the first time some of the leading audiologists in the country. Among them was Dr Kevin Murphy of the Audiology Research Unit at Reading, who invited me to come and see him when I paid my contemplated visit to the Mary Hare Grammar School at Newbury. Dr Murphy also agreed to write for me the account of the mechanism of hearing, the various causes of deafness, and what is now being done about it, that forms the appendix of this book. He was one of the 'new men' trained under Sir Alexander and Lady Ewing at the Department of Audiology and Education of the Deaf at Manchester University, which since its establishment in 1919 has been a dynamo of research into the problems of deafness, of pioneering new techniques and harnessing technological progress for the education of deaf children. A month later I visited Dr Murphy on my way to the Mary Hare Grammar School. Here I had my first glimpse of an audiology unit – that at Reading is one of the most advanced in Europe – and heard from Dr Murphy something of the new techniques for assessing the hearing of small children, of babies and even of infants in the womb (the last being still a matter of research). Here babes in arms are fitted with hearing-aids and the parents advised how best to help the development of language and speech in their deaf children. In particular I was impressed – even more than by the audiometers* and other arcane electrical contraptions – by the atmosphere of the place: cheerful, matter-of-fact, practical. For me this glimpse into the audiology unit was a glimpse of a new world.

No less so proved my visit to the Mary Hare Grammar School. Mr Askew had like Dr Murphy been trained under the Ewings at Manchester. The prospectus of the school, which he had let me have beforehand, should have prepared me. Nonetheless I found myself astonished, and becoming frankly envious, at what I saw

*An electronic device for measuring minute differences of hearing.

in the way of equipment and amenities: the chemistry and physics laboratories; the libraries (there were *two*); the domestic science classroom; the assembly hall with raised stage for acting and projector for film shows; the wood and metalwork workshops; the great sweep of the bosky park that surrounded the old manor, the new school buildings and flats for the staff; the fields for football, cricket and tennis. In the way of special equipment there were audiology rooms, while all classrooms had been fitted with group hearing-aids, none of which were available in my time. I felt like a revenant from the Stone Age. The afternoon on which I made my visit was an ordinary school working day. Mr Askew – his kindness is still on my conscience – gave up his afternoon to conducting me about the place and introducing me to the staff and pupils. More than once I was made to feel a complete ignoramus: I could only goggle at the esoteric symbols on the blackboard in the physics class. Two classes that particularly intrigued me were a class for singing and another for French. For both of these the pupils were of course using group hearing-aids. These would have been no use to me, but even without them I found myself picking up the pronunciation of the French phrases that the twelve-year-olds were repeating after their teacher, who was also requiring them to make up their own sentences in French. I was hard put to it not to join in even at the price of making a fool of myself.

All the classes were small, as is necessary in a deaf school. I was told there were about a hundred and sixty pupils of both sexes aged between eleven and eighteen. They were taught by a staff of nearly thirty full-time and part-time teachers, most with special qualifications besides being certificated teachers of the deaf. About half the pupils are partially hearing, the rest profoundly deaf – much the same proportion as at my Northampton school. I am not expert in these matters, but it seemed to me the education offered here may have been rather better than at most grammar schools in the rest of the country.

Two points were of interest to me, remembering my own schooldays: the pupils' command of language, and the amount of contact they had with the outside world. As to the first, Mr Askew placed in my hands a foolscap book, a lively handwritten account illustrated with postcards, cut-outs, and so on, of a week's sightseeing visit to London, done by one of the elder girls: done for fun, not as an exercise. Her English was not only correct; it was natural and unstilted. Afterwards I found in the school magazine, which I took away with me, poems in Scots dialect by one of the pupils. As for the second point I discovered that while some of the pupils belonged to the local troops of scouts and guides, others attended extramural classes at the Further Education College at Newbury, while there were plenty of contacts – not only games, but dances and parties – with local schools. The seniors were free to roam the countryside on foot or cycle. Mr Askew did not think they were in the least inhibited, as I had once been, when mixing with hearing people. It happened that I was able to confirm this independently. An old friend of mine, John Fairfax, who lives near Newbury, drove over to pick me up when the time came for me to leave. It turned out that he had met several of the Mary Hare sixth-formers. He pronounced them not at all shy, but very confident and lively people. They had come to one of Fairfax's poetry readings.

Mr Askew had not heard about this incident but seemed by no means surprised.

'They're very enterprising and go all over the place,' he said.

'They made one remark to me, though,' said Fairfax. 'They said they could tell that I had a deaf friend.'

'That's because I trained you to speak,' I remarked.

Having seen the audiology unit at Reading and the Mary Hare Grammar School, I came away feeling exhilarated; at the same time realizing how much my own education belonged to the pre-electronic era. Though I belong to the comparatively small category of the stone-deaf, so that I find even the more powerful of modern electronic aids useless, remarkable new devices are now being developed, known as frequency transposers, which have been found effective for people like myself. These devices are designed to harness the residuary auditory/tactile remnants; thus Dr Pierre Gorman, one of the few I have met who is as deaf as I am, has been able to differentiate clearly between sounds like 'es' and 'esh' when presented through a frequency transposer – though, having been born deaf, he had never heard either of them in his life before. I also would be able to distinguish sounds with the aid of this machine, yet although I have had seven years of hearing, that does not mean I would be able to identify words; I have been deaf too long. After forty years, it would be like learning a different language – or, more nearly, like acquiring a totally new physical skill – and would require as much intelligence and perhaps more time than I can give.

This conception of hearing as a skill lies behind the techniques of auditory training developed by the Ewings at Manchester University in the thirties. It has been made possible by technological progress in electronics which enabled ever more accurate measurements of the severity and type of hearing loss to be made, and by the appearance of more efficient and lighter transistorized hearing-aids which can even be fitted to babies. The emphasis nowadays is on the detection of deafness in children at the earliest possible moment, and the assistance and training of whatever residual hearing they may have (nearly always there is some) with the help of hearing-aids.

Not long after my visit to the Mary Hare Grammar School I spent a day at the Department of Audiology and Education of the Deaf at Manchester, where by the kindness of the head of department, Professor I. G. Taylor, and of Mrs Betty Byers Brown, the Lecturer in Speech Pathology and Therapy (whom I had met at Edinburgh, and to whom I owed my introduction) I was able to see something of the new techniques.

It was a clinic day. That morning a deaf two-year-old girl had been brought in by her mother to have the extent and nature of her hearing loss diagnosed. With older children and adults this can be done very accurately with the pure-tone audiometer. But very young infants who cannot speak or understand what is wanted of them are of course not able to tell the audiologist whether they have heard the test-sounds. However, a technique called 'play-audiometry' has been devised by which valuable information about a child's residual hearing can be obtained. It was this technique that I watched – invisible behind a one-way glass panel separating the observation-room used by students and training teachers from the audiology room where the examination was conducted. I will describe what I saw.

The tests were conducted by Professor Taylor himself and by the Lecturer in Parent Guidance, Mr Campbell. Both wore ordinary clothes; no white coats or similar hospital-paraphernalia which might upset children are permitted in the clinic. Toys are scattered about the rooms; every effort is made to put the children at ease and keep them entertained. (I thought of the alternation of boredom and fright I had undergone in consulting-rooms as a child!) The mother, a plump and attractive blonde in her late twenties, came in carrying her daughter. After a few pre-liminary questions she was seated facing Mr Campbell, with the little girl on her knee. A shelf of toys stood behind Mr Campbell, who picked up one and began talking to the child, demonstrating how it worked and capturing the little girl's attention. Mean-while Professor Taylor crept round the back of the chair in which the mother sat, holding in one hand a baby's rattle. At a moment when the little girl was wholly absorbed in Mr Campbell, the pro-fessor shook the rattle close to her ear. The child jerked her head round to the source of the noise: she had heard it. Mr Camp-bell produced a fresh toy and recaptured her attention. Now the professor tried the rattle at the other ear, and again obtained a reaction. While Mr Campbell continued to amuse the little girl Professor Taylor stealthily dodged back and forth behind her with various instruments – a whistle, a chime-bar, a bell, a cup and spoon, and so forth – to test her reaction to sounds of different pitches and frequencies. These were measured at a sound-level meter immediately afterwards. In this way a fairly detailed and accurate picture of the child's hearing capacity was built up.

In this field of 'distraction testing' Professor Taylor is a pioneer – and also a very skilled exponent; as with most things, the method is not as easy as it looks, but demands care and practice: two people have to work as a team, one holding the child's atten-tion and the other presenting the stimulus. The difficulty is to obtain exactly the right *quality* of attention from the child. If it is too engrossed, it doesn't respond to the sound; on the other hand, if its attention is allowed to wander, the head turns away from the distraction, and the child can see the movement of the instru-ment employed by the tester; in which case the response to the stimulus is equivocal – it may be response to the movement, not the sound.

Later I saw a pure-tone audiometry test being given to a boy of six or seven. The boy wore headphones through which pure tones of different pitches were passed at intervals. He sat at a table with a peg-board in front of him. The test had been turned into a game: every time the boy heard a noise through the headphones he fitted a peg into a hole. This kept the lad amused and served as a signal to the audiologist who was plotting his audiogram.

'I hope that boy isn't cheating,' I remarked.

'We provide for that by varying the intervals between the sounds,' I was told.

After the little girl had had her 'play-audiometry' (one of its purposes was to help with the prescription of the most suitable type of hearing-aid) I saw her being given an intelligence test. Here again the keynote was informality and the use of play. The tests, of course had to be non-verbal: for example, the little girl was shown how different shapes (a square, a triangle, a circle) could be fitted to their relevant places in a matrix, and then left to do it herself. These tests are designed to discover whether a child is in fact mentally retarded or deficient, as distinct from the being backward because of deafness. Both the audiometry test and intelligence tests are used to help in determining the kind of educational treatment which will best suit the child.

A baby that cannot hear well enough to distinguish words will obviously not be able to pick up understanding of language or teach itself to speak by imitation like hearing babies. Until quite recently no attempt was made to teach deaf children language or speech before they were three or four years old, if they were lucky enough to be taught at all. Now they begin as soon as a diagnosis can be made. Mr Campbell, whose task is to help and advise the parents of deaf children, told me something about it.

'We begin talking to the baby when it is seven months old,' he said.

'But what can you say to a deaf baby of seven months?' I asked rather stupidly, though truly nonplussed.

'I'll show you,' said Mr Campbell. He left the office where we were sitting and returned with a handful of toys. Picking up a ball he began talking to an imaginary baby.

'Look. This is a ball. Watch me roll the ball. Shall I roll the ball to you? Here's a cup. Now I'm going to put the ball into the cup. There! The ball is in the cup . . .'

And so he went on, fitting the action to the words, demonstrating his words by his actions. As I could see the aim was to capture the baby's interest, to familiarize it with the sound of words heard through the hearing-aid and at the time to provide the plainest clues to their meaning. Another object, he told me, was to draw attention to the movements of the face as meaningful and interesting. In this way a basis is laid for the understanding of language. The child is also being trained to listen, to use what hearing it may have. But the early grasp of language which this technique makes possible is all-important. For language is the basis of education and indeed the achievement that differentiates the human from the animal.

Yet barely four hundred years ago the deaf-born were considered ineducable and condemned, or rather abandoned, to lives negated by the lack of adequate means of communication and exchange of information. Those who became deaf in childhood were in little better case, for they either never learned to speak or reverted to inarticulacy. This glimpse of contemporary methods and techniques may serve as a gauge to the following chapters, where I propose briefly to trace the history of deafness, or rather of the rehabilitation of the deaf, from its slow and difficult beginnings to the present day. For the history of deafness is the history of the education of the deaf.

Ten

THE origins and development of the education of the deaf and dumb is an obscure but fascinating subject. Not much has been written about it.* And that history is short, for the beginnings are surprisingly recent. Not till the sixteenth century was it thought possible to teach the deaf at all. A psychological block compounded of scientific and philosophical prejudice made any attempt out of the question. People took it for granted that it was impossible for deaf mutes to learn to speak or understand language, or even – in the words of a Commission of Inquiry set up by the French Academy of Sciences in 1749 – 'become capable of reasoning and acting like others'.

Why this should have been so can be understood if one ponders the effect of deafness at birth or in early childhood. At this stage of life it is a calamity worse than blindness, because the consequences strike at the roots of intellectual development. Loss of hearing involves loss of the only means by which a child acquires language. 'The blind man goes to school in his cradle,' as George Dalgarno, an early pioneer of the education of the deaf,

---

* The earliest historical survey of deafness is found in Hervas y Panduro's *Escuela española de sordomudos* (1795) and in Baron Degerando's *De l'Éducation des sourds-muets de naissance* (1827). But of more recent work a good account is contained in *The Story of Lipreading: Its Genesis and Development*, by Fred DeLand (1931) while Dr Ruth E. Bender's *The Conquest of Deafness*, The Press of Case-Western Reserve University (1960), is more up to date and comprehensive. Very interesting and valuable accounts are contained in D. G. Pritchard's *Education and the Handicapped*, Routledge; New York: Humanities Press (1963) and particularly in Kenneth W. Hodgson's *The Deaf and Their Problems* (1953). Thomas Arnold's *Education of Deaf Mutes: A Manual for Teachers* (1888, and subsequent editions) contains an invaluable Historical Introduction to which Arnold's pupil, Abraham Farrar, contributed much research. The latest edition of Farrar's revised and rewritten version of Arnold's book came out in 1954 (*Arnold on the Education of the Deaf*). The best survey of recent developments is undoubtedly Thomas J. Watson's *The Education of Hearing-handicapped Children*, University of London Press; Illinois: Charles C. Thomas (1967). To the last six books the present account is greatly indebted.

pointed out in the seventeenth century. For the blind can at least hear, and so pick up speech and language like other children. But the deaf child, left to his own resources, must grow up not only unable to speak but denied even a concept of language, that indispensable instrument of thinking and reasoning. Not only is he unable to communicate with others, he cannot even communicate with himself – he has no language with which to think about what he sees and experiences. Thus, unable to receive or transmit any but the most elementary communications by means of signs, with his reasoning faculty atrophied or badly hampered for lack of a vehicle, a deaf-born person may grow up indistinguishable from an idiot. His case is worse, for his is not a defective but a trapped and frustrated intelligence. The effect of deafness at birth is to turn its victim into a Caliban.

When Prospero met Caliban:

> I pitied thee,
> Took pains to make thee speak, taught thee each hour
> One thing or other. When thou didst not, savage,
> Know thine own meaning, but wouldst gabble like
> A thing most brutish, I endow'd thy purposes
> With words that made them known.

Yet the words of Shakespeare – 'took pains to make thee speak' embody what was, even in the seventeenth century, a new concept: the notion that speech, instead of being a natural instinct or function, is in fact an acquired art and therefore teachable. Until this idea had become current no one understood that the dumbness of the deaf-born was a *result* of deafness, and not a concomitant disability. And in fact it was in Shakespeare's lifetime that the deaf found their Prospero: a Spanish Benedictine monk Pedro Ponce de León. It is most unlikely that Shakespeare ever heard of him; yet Prospero's methods with Caliban – 'taught thee each hour One thing or other', 'endow'd thy purposes With words that made them known' – seem a fair approximation to those of Ponce de León, the first man, so far as is known, to teach deaf mutes to speak.

Why was it that, up to the time of Pedro Ponce de León – he died in 1584 – the deaf and dumb had been abandoned to their helpless and hopeless condition, bracketed with infants and the insane by the law, and regarded by doctors and philosophers as incurable and unteachable? Part of the reason, ironically, was

that the terrible and repellent consequences of their disability –
uncouthness, animality, uncomprehendingness and incomprehensibility – were not those which inspire sympathy. Antiquity tells
of blind poets, blind prophets and seers, of lame gods and kings
and saints, but of no deaf mutes – certainly not in these categories. In nearly every language the word 'dumb' has the connotation 'stupid'.*

Another factor was the way in which the few and mostly
unhelpful references to deafness in the works of the early philosophers and scientists tended to become a basis of prejudice.
When Aristotle, in his *History of Animals*, made the factual observation 'Those who are born deaf all become speechless, they
have a voice, but are destitute of speech' (*Hist. anim.* IV. ix)
word ' ἐνεοὶ' (speechless, could also be taken in the sense of
'stupid') and the sentence, quoted out of its context, could be and
was interpreted to mean that the deaf-born become imbecile.
Pliny the Elder, the Roman polymath who perished in the eruption that destroyed Pompeii, remarked in his *Natural History*
'There are no persons born deaf that are not also dumb.' True
enough; yet this was taken to point to a physical and not a consequential link between deafness and dumbness, which was elaborated by Galen a century after Pliny. Galen (*c.* A.D. 130-200) who
was regarded as the greatest of physicians after Hippocrates, put
forward the theory of a common cerebral origin of speech and
hearing, by which damage to the one must involve damage to the
other. Speech and hearing were inseparable. It followed that deaf
mutes could not be taught to articulate. Such authoritative dicta
(and it must be remembered that up to the sixteenth century the
affirmations of people like Aristotle and even Galen were almost
as unchallengeable as Holy Writ) helped to establish an accepted
opinion that dumbness and cretinism were physical adjuncts of
congenital deafness rather than its consequences. Everything
pointed to the conclusion that deaf mutes were ineducable, that
for them nothing could be done.

* In parenthesis, the prestige of speech is symbolized in the hierarchy of
the priesthood of the Mlimo cult in Mashonaland (present-day Rhodesia).
The Mlimo, or oracular god, was served by three officers of ascending rank:
Maziso (The Eye), to whom reports were made, Nzewe (The Ear) to whom
petitions were addressed, and Murumo (The Mouth), chief priest of the cult,
through whom the oracle spoke. This may point to the relative importance of the faculties of sight, hearing, and language in the eyes of primitive
people.

And nothing was done, or almost nothing. In the earliest times the Jews and to some extent the Egyptians and Persians treated their deaf-born humanely compared with the ancient Greeks and Romans; at least they were permitted to live and even given some protection by law. But the Athenians and Spartans exposed or killed malformed or crippled babies, while the early Roman practice was to destroy children at the age of three if they seemed likely to prove a liability to the community. Many deaf-born infants may have been accounted for by these customs, though a good few must have escaped because deafness is not easy to detect in babies. Apart from the Mosaic negative injunction 'Thou shalt not curse the deaf' almost the only mention of them in antiquity is the miracle recounted by St Mark. He relates how Christ restored to a deaf mute – in a perhaps significant order – hearing and then speech. That the bystanders 'were beyond measure astonished, saying "He hath done all things well: he maketh both the deaf to hear, and the dumb to speak" ' may suggest the hopelessness with which their condition was regarded.

Writing in the nineteenth century, Thomas Arnold suggested that the very absence of reference to the deaf and dumb in classical times might be taken to point to the wretched existence they must have endured. 'Their presence in the family was felt to be a disgrace and calamity. Destitute of education, and hardly understood, even in expressing their wants by signs, they lived in deplorable isolation, looked upon as useless, a burden ... No other class suffered so much.'* This however seems assumption, for nothing is certainly known about their treatment. My own feeling is that Arnold may have been drawing on his experience of the institutions in which the industrial revolution herded and segregated the deaf-mute children of the masses (as a young man he had taught in one of them and been horrified by it) and supposed that the condition of the deaf must have been similar, or worse, in the pre-Christian era. But around 70 B.C. we hear of one M. V. Corvinus, an orator, who is said to have had a deaf and dumb relative instructed in painting. Some half a century later there was the similar case, recorded by Pliny in his *Natural History*, of Quintus Pedius, the first deaf mute whose name has come down to us. He was the son of that Quintus Pedius who was a Roman Consul and co-heir of the emperor Augustus. With the approval of Augustus, so Pliny says, Quintus Pedius was taught to paint –

* Thomas Arnold, *Education of Deaf-Mutes* (1888).

an experiment which proved successful. This initiates a pattern: until the eighteenth century the few deaf mutes to receive instruction were nearly always children of the rich and powerful. Even today it is only the richer countries that can afford to do much about the education of their deaf children.

Seven centuries go by before we come upon the next instance – Bede's account of St John of Beverley teaching a dumb youth to speak. In the first part of this book I have quoted the passage describing this 'miracle'. Bede does not say the lad could not hear, but it seems likely, to judge from the technique employed by St John – at any rate he is regarded as a patron saint of teachers of the deaf on the strength of it.* Not for eight hundred years after Bede wrote his *History of the English Church* is there mention of a deaf man. In 1528 appeared a posthumously published book, *De Inventione Dialectica*, the work of a Dutch scholar called Rodolphus Agricola of Groningen, who died in 1485. Among other things Agricola spoke of a deaf mute who had learned to read and write. This story was sceptically commented on by Ludovic Vives, a famous Spanish scholar, educationalist, and friend of Erasmus:

The sense of hearing teaches both more and greater things and more quickly ... nor has Aristotle undeservedly named this the sense of education; living things deprived of it are not capable of education. Wherefore the more wonder that there was one born deaf and dumb, who had learned letters, as R. Agricola, who has related this, observes.

Hearing, especially before the invention of printing, was almost the only medium of instruction, hence the polite incredulity that Vives expressed at Agricola's story. As Farrar remarked, 'the essentially artificial nature of speech was not realized, and the possibility of there being other avenues to the mind was either only dimly or not at all perceived ... Speech being the recognized medium of education, the absence of this faculty implied the exclusion of deaf mutes from intellectual instruction.'† But the tide was turning, and Agricola's deaf mute helped to turn it.

The *De Inventione Dialectica* came into the hands of one Girolamo Cardano, an Italian physician, mathematician, astronomer, and astrologer, who has been described as 'the first psychologist'. Born in 1501, Cardano was one of the liveliest speculative

* Tradition says that this story of Bede's inspired Ponce de León to attempt teaching the deaf.

† Juan Pablo Bonet, *Method of Teaching Deaf Mutes to Speak*, translated by H. N. Dixon, Historical Introduction by A. Farrar (1890).

thinkers of the Renaissance. Like his contemporary Benvenuto Cellini he wrote an entertaining autobiography, *De Vita Propria Libre*, which some have seen as a forerunner of Rousseau's *Confessions*, for in this book he examined himself 'as if he were a new species of animal which he never expected to see again'. Cardano's eldest son was deaf in one ear, and he himself was afflicted with a stutter. These chances, as so often in the history of deafness, may have led him to take interest in the problem, though he speculated nearly always perceptively and usefully, about almost every subject under the sun: he was one of the first to suggest that the blind might be taught to read and write through the sense of touch. Cardano's positive response to the story of the literate deaf mute was in complete contrast to the negative reaction of the orthodox Vives. For the conclusions that Cardano drew from it dissolved the block that made education of the deaf appear impossible.

Agricola relates ... that he had seen a man born deaf and dumb, who had learned to read and write, so that he could express whatever he wished. Thus it is possible to place a deaf mute in a position to hear by reading, and to speak by writing; for his memory leads him to understand, by reflection, that *bread*, as written, signifies the thing which is eaten. He thus reads, by the light of his reason as it were, in a picture; for by this means, though nothing is referred to sounds, not only objects but actions and results are made known. And just as after seeing a picture, we may draw another picture, guided simply by a conception of the objects represented, such is also the case with letters. For as different sounds are conventionally used to signify different things, so also may the various figures of objects and words.

Paralipomena

That is to say one sense can be substitute for another: if the deaf cannot hear, they can see, and if they can see, they can learn to read; in the same way, if they cannot speak, they can learn to write. For Cardano grasped the elementary proposition that 'writing is associated with speech and speech with thought; but written characters and ideas may be connected without the intervention of actual sounds'. This seems obvious enough, but in the sixteenth century the notion that the understanding of ideas did not depend on the hearing of words was revolutionary. The education of the deaf had been made theoretically possible: Cardano's premise became the principle upon which it was based.

Yet Cardano does not seem to have put his ideas into practice

– at any rate there is no record of his having taught the deaf. Nevertheless before Cardano died in 1576 Ponce de León was not only teaching deaf mutes to read and write but, to the astonishment of all who heard of it, to speak as well.

Pedro Ponce de León was born at Valladolid about 1520. He graduated at the university of Salamanca before becoming a monk at the Benedictine monastery of San Salvador at Oña near Burgos. His interest in the deaf seems to have arisen through personal contact. There was one Gaspard Burgos who wished to enter the monastery of San Salvador as a convert but, being deaf and dumb, was debarred – not being able to speak he could not make confession. Ponce de León is said to have become interested in the man and successfully taught him to write and speak. The story is not well authenticated, but there is no doubt about his success with other deaf-mute pupils. They were not obscure postulants like Gaspard Burgos, but scions of the noblest families in Spain.

It was not entirely accidental that in the sixteenth century Spain should have been the country where the education of the deaf was first attempted and encouraged. Spain was then at the zenith of her wealth and power. The discovery and exploitation of the Americas had won her immense riches, which had mostly found their way into the hands of a comparatively few noble families. At the same time Spanish society remained almost anachronistically feudal and stratified. The aristocratic exclusiveness of these families inclined them to frequent intermarriages, occassionally resulting in the birth of congenitally deaf children who were often sole heirs of great estates. According to the Spanish legal code, which was based on Roman Law, deaf and dumb persons were legally incapable – that is, they could not own property or make wills.* This meant that should the heir of an estate be

* The history of the legal position of the deaf begins with Jewish Law. The Talmud discriminated between deaf mutes and those who were deaf only and dumb only. Deaf mutes were held to be incapable of owning property; their legal status was that of children. Those who could speak but not hear, and those who could hear but not speak, were accorded certain rights. Roman Law took over and developed the Talmudic discrimination between grades of deafness. Thus the Code of Justinian recognized five separate classes, of which only the first – those deaf and dumb from birth – was completely without rights and obligations: they could neither own property nor enter into contracts. But the deaf who could speak were regarded as persons at law, who could own property, marry, make wills. These laws and distinctions found their way into most legal codes based on Roman Law.

deaf and dumb he could not inherit; the estate and title must pass to the next of kin. This was the dilemma of more than one wealthy family in sixteenth-century Spain. But if the deaf-mute heir could be taught to speak, it followed that his legal disability would be nullified. This proved a powerful stimulus to encouraging any method of educating deaf mutes.

The motives of Ponce de León were primarily religious, but it is not surprising to find that his deaf-mute pupils were all heirs of noble and wealthy families. Nor is it surprising that when he died in 1584 his work and methods should have been continued and developed by others under the patronage of the Spanish ruling classes.* Ponce de León's two most famous pupils were Francisco and Pedro de Velasco, deaf and dumb brothers, relatives of the Constable of Castile. Pedro de Velasco appears to have been an intelligent and attractive character who learned to speak well enough to take up the privileges and duties he had inherited, including military service. According to Velasco, Ponce de León taught the brothers to read, write, and speak; they were able to make spoken confessions, pray, and assist at Mass. A witness† speaks of hearing Pedro de Velasco singing the plain chant, the

* Yet it must not be supposed that all deaf mutes remained morons. Ponce de León, so far as we know, was the first systematic instructor of the deaf, and the first to teach articulation, but there were cases of exceptionally intelligent or exceptionally lucky deaf mutes who, like the one mentioned by Agricola, progressed as far as reading and writing. Early in the sixteenth century Oecolampadius, the friend and coadjutor of Martin Luther, is said to have taught a deaf boy to read, and another Lutheran clergyman, Joachim Pasch, to have instructed his deaf daughter by means of pictures. And there was a famous deaf and dumb contemporary of Ponce de León's, the Spanish painter Juan Fernández Navarette, called 'El Mudo'. He was taught to paint at the monastery of L'Étoile, sent to Italy to study under Titian, and became painter to Philip II: his work is still to be seen in the Escorial. It is said El Mudo was able to explain himself by signs, could read, write, and play cards. When he died at Toledo in 1579 his epitaph was written by Lope de Vega. The following is a prose translation:

Heaven denied me speech, that by my understanding I might give greater feeling to the things which I painted; and such great life did I give them with my skilful pencil, that as I could not speak I made them speak for me.

† The licentiate Lasso, a contemporary of Ponce de Léon's, whose manuscript account of his achievements in teaching Pedro and Francisco de Velasco was written at the monastery of Oña in 1550 and has been called the earliest treatise on the education of the deaf; though it is really an exposition of the legal rights and status of Francisco de Velasco after he had been taught to speak. Pedro de Velasco's account of his education, quoted below, appears in this manuscript.

choir following him and helping him to keep tune and time. Ponce de León claimed that he taught some of his pupils Latin, Greek, and Italian besides their own language – but perhaps that was laying it on a bit. He is said to have left a record of his technique, but it was lost, probably in the fire that burned the monastery library. It would appear that he followed Cardano's suggested method, first teaching his pupils language by associating written words with the objects they signified. That achieved, he was able to begin to teach them to articulate. For religious reasons speech was his chief aim, as for legal and economic motives it was that of his employers. How far he succeeded may be gauged from Pedro de Velasco's rather charming account:

When I was a child I knew nothing, like a stone; but I commenced to learn by first of all writing down the things my master taught me ... Then next, by the aid of God, I began to spell, and afterwards to pronounce with all the force I could, although much saliva came from me. After this I began to read histories, so that in ten years I had read the histories of the whole of the world; and then I learnt Latin.

After the death of Ponce de León his work was carried on by Manuel Ramírez de Carrión and Juan Pablo Bonet. Bonet, a soldier and a man of affairs, was born in 1579. He became secretary to another Constable of Castile, a great-nephew of the pupils of Ponce de León. This Constable's younger brother, Luis de Velasco, the Marquis of Fresno, was a deaf mute like his great-uncles; as so often, deafness ran in the family. Both Bonet and Carrión had a hand in teaching this young man, though the details are uncertain. Probably Bonet undertook his education in the first place and then, owing to the pressure of his other duties, employed Carrión to continue it. The latter seems to have been an excellent practical teacher of the deaf, for he afterwards took on other pupils including the Marquis de Priego and Prince Emmanuel of Savoy. In 1629 Carrión published a book called *Maravillas de naturaleza* in which he boasted of having taught the deaf and dumb to speak; without, however, revealing his methods. As we shall discover, this secretiveness was to be characteristic of many teachers of the deaf till well into the nineteenth century. So, perhaps, was jealousy: for though both Carrión and Bonet wrote about teaching the deaf, neither mentions the other, nor even Ponce de León, to whose work and example they must have owed much.

To Bonet belongs the credit of publishing in 1620 the first treatise on the education of the deaf, *Reducción de las letras, y arte* *para enseñar a hablar los mudos* (Simplification of the Letters of the Alphabet and Method of Teaching Deaf Mutes to Speak). This enormously important book is a landmark – 'the literary foundation stone of deaf education'.* The first part is concerned with a system of associating letters of the alphabet with their phonetic elements in order to simplify reading. Here Bonet may be said to anticipate modern ideas. His attempt to posit an analogy between the shapes of the letters of the alphabet and their articulation (for instance, he takes the letter B to represent the closed position of the lips when making the sound) may be claimed as a forerunner of Bell's 'Visible Speech' (see note, p. 153). The second part details a method of teaching deaf mutes language and speech which is basically still in use; it probably derived from the one evolved by Ponce de León. To begin with Bonet advocated the teaching of a one-handed manual alphabet (still in use in America) in association with the printed one. He insisted that everyone in contact with the pupil should learn and use this alphabet, and avoid resort to signs when speaking with him, as the best way of making him learn words and language. Next the pupil was taught to pronounce letters, beginning with vowels, which are the easiest; then syllables, then words: finally he was taught his own native language by set grammatical steps. Bonet realized that all intellectual development depends on language and used every means of encouraging its acquisition. As an exercise in the use of language, he laid down that 'it will be an important part of his [the pupil's] education that he be asked every evening what he has done in the daytime'. He stressed the importance of making the pupil read books, and of written exercises. He noted the value of lipreading, though he did not think it could be taught systematically. Though many of Bonet's principles and techniques were independently rediscovered by later teachers, what Bonet did was to clear the way for his successors; and his treatise influenced, if only by hearsay, all who came after him.

The Spanish achievement in educating the deaf became known through an eyewitness account by that odd fish, Sir Kenelm Digby. The son of one of the Gunpowder Plot conspirators, Digby

---

* Kenneth W. Hodgson, *The Deaf and Their Problems*. Bonet's book, however, was not the first monograph on deafness; that distinction probably belongs to a book called *Oratio de surditate et mutitate*, by Salomon Alberti of Nuremberg, which came out in 1591. This was largely a medical work, though Alberti discusses lipreading as a phenomenon.

was by turns diplomat, privateer, philosopher, autobiographer, and poet. 'I have seen one who could discern sounds with his eyes,' Digby related among other marvels in his *Treatise on the Nature of Bodies* (1644), written while he was in exile in Paris. He went on to recount the unprecedented accomplishments of a deaf mute he had known: none other than the deaf-born brother of the Constable of Castile, whom he and Charles I of England had met twenty years before. This was the Marquis of Fresno, the pupil of Carrión and Bonet. In 1623 Charles I, then Prince of Wales, was at Madrid with the Duke of Buckingham on an abortive mission, part serious, part escapade, to win the hand of the Infanta. Digby, whose uncle was English Ambassador at Madrid, had contrived to join the party. While there Digby became acquainted with the deaf Marquis:

The Spanish lord was borne deafe . . . and consequently he was dumbe; for not being able to heare the sound of words he could neither imitate nor understand them. The lovelinesse of his face and especially the exceeding life and spiritfulnesse of his eyes, and the comelinesse of his person and whole composure of his body throughout, were pregnant figures of a well-tempered mind within . . . Att the last, there was a priest who undertook the teaching him to understand others when they spoke, and to speake himself that others might understand him. What att the first he was laught att for made him after some yeares to be looked upon as if he had wrought a miracle. In a word after strange patience, constancy and paines, he brought the yong Lord to speake as distinctly as any man whosoever . . . They who have a curiosity to see by what steppes the master proceeded in teaching him, may satisfy it by a booke which he himself hath writ in Spanish upon that subject, to instruct others how to teach deafe and dumbe persons to speake . . .

The 'priest' to whom Digby refers may possibly have been Bonet, though he does not mention his name. At any rate Digby introduced the deaf Marquis to his royal master, who seems to have taken a great interest in him. The young man could, says Digby,

repeat after any body, any hard word whatsoever. Which the Prince tryed often; not only in English, but by making some Welchmen that served his Highnesse, speake wordes of their language. Which he so perfectly echoed, that I confesse I wondered more att that, than att all the rest.

The feat does sound incredible, and was indeed received with scepticism by at least one of Digby's seventeenth-century readers; but it is a trick well within the compass of an adequately taught and adept deaf person. The exactness and trustworthiness of Digby's observation is shown by his description of the Marquis's lipreading:

the knowledge he had of what they said sprung from his observing the motions they made; so that he could converse currently in the light, though they they talked with whispered never so softly. And I have seene him at the distance of a large chamber's breadth say wordes after one, that I standing close by the speaker could not heare a syllable of. But if he were in the darke, or if one turned his face out of his sight, he was capable of nothing one said.

It was to be another two centuries before the education of the deaf and dumb began to be generally undertaken. But in the hundred years since Cardano the crucial advance had been made. Cardano scotched the accepted opinion that the deaf and dumb were incapable of education. Ponce de León and his successors furnished practical proof that Cardano was right. In demonstrating that deaf mutes could be taught language, and even articulation, the Spanish pioneers had achieved a breakthrough that shattered for ever the old assumptions on the nature of deafness and speech. It was a psychological turning-point like the rounding of Cape Bojador, which in the previous century had opened the way to the finding of the sea-route to India and the discovery of the Americas. (Cape Bojador, supposed to mark the end of the world where the waters of the ocean poured over the earth's rim into the abyss, had been doubled by Henry the Navigator's famous captain, Gil Eannes, in 1434. Once this had been done the myth was exploded, and the voyages of Columbus and Vasco da Gama made possible.) But unlike the sea-route to the Indies the problems of the deaf were unromantic, obscure, and of no pressing moment for most people. Thus no great notice was taken of the achievements of Ponce de León or his successors.* Not until the publication of Digby's book in 1644 was the work of the Spanish teachers made known in England, where already a Dr John Bulwer, who was to be the first to advocate 'an academy for the mute', had been interesting himself in the problems of the deaf.

*At least Cervantes heard of them; for in one of his stories, *El licenciado vidriera*, published 1614, he mentions a monk who taught the dumb to speak – possibly a reference to Ponce.

Eleven

THE seventeenth century was a time of wide-ranging intellectual and scientific curiosity and activity. In Britain it was the age of Bacon, Newton, Boyle, Hobbes, Locke, and Harvey, besides any number of agile and inquiring minds like Sir Kenelm Digby, Sir Christopher Wren, Robert Hooke, and Newton's precursor, the mathematician Dr John Wallis. The latter, who played an important role in the history of deaf education, was one of the founders of the Royal Society, which began as a sort of scientific debating club. Among other things, the symbolic nature of language began to intrigue and preoccupy a surprising number of seventeenth-century intellectuals. As will be seen, from the nature of language to the nature of communication, thence to the practical problems of the deaf and dumb, was a natural progression for many. Thus, in the same year that Digby's *Treatise on the Nature of Bodies* appeared, a Dr John Bulwer published a curious monograph on the use and value of manual gestures for speech, oratory and acting, entitled *Chirologia: or the Naturall Language of the Hand*. In the course of his book Dr Bulwer mentioned 'one Master Babington of Burntwood in the County of Essex', a deaf man who 'doth notwithstanding feele words and, as if he had an eye in his finger, sees signs in the dark; whose wife discourseth very perfectly with him by a strange way of arthrologie, or alphabet contrived on the joynts of his fingers; who taking him by the hand in the night, can so discourse with him very exactly'.

In parenthesis, it is a remarkable fact that systems of finger-spelling and expressive formal gesture were in existence long before there was any idea of using them as a means of communication for the deaf. The ancient Greeks had a system of numeration by the fingers from which the earliest finger alphabets may have derived. Between the second and fourth centuries A.D. the art of signing was brought to perfection by the actors of the Roman *pantomimi*, a kind of ballet-mime that had supplanted the true drama. Manual alphabets were used by monastic orders, particularly those bound to silence like the Cistercians. In his *De loquela* *per gestum digitorum* the Venerable Bede refers to three different forms which must have been in existence before the eighth century. And the underworld found a use for finger-spelling as a silent and safer kind of 'flash' or argot for secret communication.* Yet so far as is known Ponce de León and Bonet were the first to use a manual alphabet for the deaf. Bonet's treatise on deaf education contains an engraved illustration of the system he employed. It is the one-hand manual alphabet still current in America, but cannot have been the invention of either Bonet or Ponce de León, for it is to be found in Rossellius's *Artificiosae memoriae*, published at Venice in 1579, half a century before the appearance of Bonet's treatise. Indeed the first finger alphabet invented specifically for the deaf did not appear till 1680, in George Dalgarno's *Deaf and Dumb Man's Tutor*. The earliest version of the two-handed finger alphabet now generally used first appeared in 1698, in a pamphlet called *Digiti-Lingua*.

It was not with the deaf in mind that Dr Bulwer had written the *Chirologia*, though he was soon to take an interest in them.

From Digby's *Treatise on the Nature of Bodies* Bulwer learned of the work of the Spanish teachers of the deaf. Four years later, in 1648, he brought out the first English work on deafness, dedicated to Sir Edward Gosticke, a deaf and dumb gentleman who communicated by signs and finger-spelling, but desired to learn to speak. *Philocophus: or the Deafe and Dumbe Mans Friend* sets out to prove 'That a Man borne Deafe and Dumbe, may be taught to Heare the sound of *wordes* with his *Eie*, & thence learne to speake with his Tongue.' Besides a commentary on Digby's account of the deaf Spanish lord, it contains a valuable discussion of the possibility of educating deaf mutes, as well as original and percipient observations on lipreading (which Bulwer calls 'lip grammar' or 'the art of Labiall Augurie'). Yet, as in the case of Girolamo Cardano, there is no direct evidence that Bulwer put his ideas into practice.

Very soon a far more eminent savant than the comparatively obscure Dr Bulwer began to interest himself in the education of the deaf. This was Dr John Wallis, who for more than half a century held the chair of geometry at Oxford. Wallis had been born in 1616. During the Civil War he made practical use of his

* Even today the diamond merchants of Hatton Garden who do business in the street use a secret manual code. And anyone who has been to a race-course must have seen the tic-tac men signalling the odds.

mathematic bent by decoding Royalist despatches in cipher for the Parliamentarians. Though best known for pioneer work on the calculus, and for a long and bitter mathematical controversy with the philosopher Thomas Hobbes (who, not being in the same class as a mathematician, had the worst of it), Wallis was also interested in language. In 1653 he published an English grammar to which he added an essay on phonetics. He corresponded with Sir Kenelm Digby, and learned from him of Bonet's work: a circumstance which, together with his interest in phonetics, may have led him to make the practical experiment of attempting to teach a deaf mute to speak. An unusual undertaking for a professor of geometry, but in accord with the pragmatical and enterprising spirit of the seventeenth-century schoolmen. In 1661 Wallis began the instruction of 'one Mr Daniel Whalley of Northampton' who had become deaf at the age of five. A year later he was able to produce his pupil before the newly founded Royal Society and demonstrate his ability to pronounce words.

Yet Wallis was not the first English teacher of the deaf, though he claimed to be. For in 1659 another Fellow of the Royal Society, Dr William Holder,* had begun the education of a deaf-born child, Alexander Popham, a relation of the Earl of Oxford. Dr Holder, though ingenious (he used a leather strap to illustrate the position of the tongue in the articulation of various sounds) seems not to have been very successful with Popham. But it should be remembered that Popham, being born deaf, must have been a harder proposition than Whalley, who would have had some remembrance of language. Popham's mother removed him from Dr Holder and sent him to the apparently more efficacious Dr Wallis. The transfer of Popham to Dr Wallis was not well taken by Dr Holder, and even less Dr Wallis's boast that he was first in the field. It led to a violent and interminable public squabble between the two savants. But this academic row did something to publicize the fact that the education of the deaf was no longer an impossibility.

Both the learned doctors published accounts of their methods. Holder's *Elements of Speech*, with an *Appendix concerning Persons Deaf and Dumb*, appeared in 1669 and describes his system for teaching Alexander Popham. Wallis gave details of his

* Holder (1615–98), an Oxfordshire clergyman, married a sister of Sir Christopher Wren, who, incidentally, is said to have invented a manual alphabet – perhaps for Holder?

own methods in letters to Robert Boyle and Thomas Beverley which were published in the Royal Society's *Philosophical Transactions* for July 1670 and October 1698. Holder, despite his failure with Popham, was the better phonetician and more interested in teaching articulation than Wallis, whose emphasis was on the teaching of language by means of writing, the manual alphabet, lists of names of objects, and finally syntax; articulation he taught separately, and sometimes not at all. Essentially the methods of both Holder and Wallis were a rediscovery of those of Bonet and Ponce de León.

The work of George Dalgarno, a friend and contemporary of Wallis, was more forward-looking though it never achieved anything like the same celebrity. Born at Aberdeen in about 1626 he taught at a grammar school in Oxford and was another of the many seventeenth-century intellectuals who speculated on the nature of language. His first book, *Ars Signorum*,* published in 1661, was an attempt to provide a system of characters to represent ideas, not words, so that they could be read in any language. Like Bulwer and Wallis, Dalgarno's interest in the symbolism of language led him to consider the problems of the deaf, and like them he heard of Bonet through Sir Kenelm Digby. In 1680 Dalgarno published his *Didiascalocophus: Or the Deaf and Dumb Mans Tutor*. This introduced an ingenious manual alphabet of his own, the first to be invented specifically for the deaf. But Dalgarno's real contribution lay in adapting the ideas of Comenius,† the great educational reformer, to the teaching of the deaf. In contrast to the rigid learning-by-rote formula of the medieval educationalists, Comenius saw that we learn from what we see around us and that the teaching of words and things must go together. He was the first to produce an educational picture-book for children, and his revolutionary theories heralded those of Pestalozzi and Froebel. Thus Dalgarno, in his *Didiascalocophus*, was far ahead of Wallis in psychological understanding and educational theory when he advocated teaching the deaf child thus:

* The Art of Signs: a Universal Alphabet and a Philosophic Language', to give it its full title in English.

† John Amos Komensky, or Comenius, born 1592 in Moravia and died at Amsterdam in 1670. The Swedish statesman Oxenstierna invited him to Sweden to reorganize and reform its educational system. Comenius's principal work was *The Great Didactic*, written in Czech but published in a Latin translation in 1657.

Imitate the way of the nursery. Let utile and jucundum (use and joy) invite and spur him on . . . You must not be too grammatical in teaching till you find his capacity will bear it. He must not be dealt with like schoolboys, who are often punished for not learning what is above their capacity. It is enough for him to understand the word or sentence proposed, without parsing every word or syllable; for this is all the use of language that not only he but even people of age, that are illiterate, have.

But it was not until the nineteenth century that these ideas were to be revived and put in practice.

Seventeen years after the death of Dr Wallis in 1703 the problems of deafness and the feasibility of educating deaf mutes was brought to the notice of a more general public. In 1720, the year following the appearance of *Robinson Crusoe*, Daniel Defoe made a deaf mute the hero of one of his documentary novels – *The Life and Adventures of Mr Duncan Campbell*. This Duncan Campbell really existed; Steele and Addison had written of him in the *Spectator* (Nos. 474 and 560), and he was still alive when Defoe's book came out, for he did not die till 1730. According to Defoe's account Campbell had been born deaf and taught language by Dr Wallis's method, though he never attained articulation. Society was less interested in Duncan Campbell's attainments as a deaf mute than in his supposed talents as a seer and fortune-teller: most of Defoe's novel has to do with this aspect of his hero, with the evidence and arguments for and against the existence of the supernatural, magic, witchcraft, second-sight, and what would nowadays be called extra-sensory perception. But the opening chapters of his novel contain a lucid summary of the problems of the deaf and of teaching language to the deaf-born. Dr Wallis's system is described in detail, even to the printing of a long excerpt from one of Wallis's pamphlets – 'This extract is mostly taken out of the ingenious Dr Wallis, and lying hid in that little book, which is but rarely inquired after, and too scarcely known, died, in a manner, with that great man.' An engraved illustration of the two-handed finger alphabet – almost the same as that used today – provided a frontispiece. Defoe's novel was the first popular exposé of the problems of the deaf and of a method for their education.

One reader of Defoe's novel was to become the first professional teacher of the deaf in England. The eighteenth century began with the emergence of professional teachers of the deaf in Britain and on the Continent, who were as much activated by the desire, or need, to make a living from their skill as by the disinterested scientific curiosity of seventeenth-century pioneers like Wallis and Dalgarno; and it was to end with the founding of the first deaf schools. In England the first professional teacher was the naturalist Henry Baker, born in 1698 and like Wallis and Holder Fellow of the Royal Society. When a young man he visited a relation at Enfield whose eight-year-old daughter turned out to be deaf and dumb. Baker convinced himself that he could teach her language and speech. About this time Defoe's book appeared and very likely introduced Baker to the work of Dr Wallis. In any case Baker made Defoe's acquaintance (later he married Defoe's youngest daughter Sophia). Meanwhile Baker's tuition of his first pupil, Jane Forster, proved so effective that he began to take on others. He was able to command a good fee for his services, and came to depend on his teaching for a large part of his livelihood. For this reason he was secretive about his methods. He even exacted securities of as much as £100 from his pupils not to disclose them. Those he undertook to teach were carefully chosen, for he would not attempt to educate anyone unless he felt sure of success – failure would be a bad advertisement. Not a great deal is known of Baker's method, but he claimed to have improved Dr Wallis's system and seems to have been far more successful than he in teaching articulation. In any case the specialized techniques evolved for teaching the deaf were regarded as professional secrets by those who, like Baker, made it their living. This was certainly true of the famous Braidwood dynasty, which for nearly sixty years was to hold a virtual monopoly of the education of the deaf in Britain.

When Dr Samuel Johnson wrote his *Journey to the Western Islands of Scotland* (1775) he elected to close it with an account of what he considered one of the more remarkable curiosities he had come across in his travels. It was, he implied, the most notable the capital of Scotland had to offer; one which 'no other city has to show; a college of the deaf and dumb, who are taught to speak, to read, to write, and to practise arithmetic, by a gentleman whose name is Braidwood. The number that attends him is, I think, about twelve . . .' The dictionary-maker was able to praise their accuracy in spelling, noting shrewdly that this was a result of learning to write before learning to speak. 'For letters to them are not symbols of names, but of things; when they write they do not represent a sound, but delineate a form.'* The proficiency of the pupils at lipreading seems to have impressed Dr Johnson most: 'They not only speak, write, and understand what is written, but if he that speaks looks towards them, and modifies his organs by distinct and full utterance, they know so well what is spoken, that it is an expression scarcely figurative to say, they hear with the eye.' And he wound up with one of his usual cracks at Caledonia: 'It was pleasing to see one of the most desperate of human calamities capable of so much help; whatever enlarges hope will exalt courage; after seeing the deaf taught arithmetic, who would be afraid to cultivate the Hebrides?'

The Braidwood Academy at Edinburgh, the first deaf school in Britain, had begun in 1760 with one pupil. By the time Dr Johnson published this report of his visit, Braidwood and his school were already famous, the subject of an article in the *Encyclopedia Britannica*, of an account in Lord Monboddo's *Of the Origin and Progress of Language*, and of some glowing pages in Thomas Pennant's *Tour in Scotland*. The headmaster of the Academy, Thomas Braidwood, had been born in 1715. He had taken a degree at Edinburgh University, later becoming proprietor of a mathematical school in that city. Chance turned him into a teacher of the deaf when in 1760 he was asked to take on a lad called Charles Shirreff who had lost his hearing at the age of three. Braidwood had neither experience nor theoretical knowledge of teaching the deaf, but thought he could make a success of Shirreff. He succeeded by dint of patience, ingenuity, and indefatigability. Like all the greatest teachers of the deaf, Braidwood had an intuitive genius for the work. He read up Bulwer, Wallis, and Holder, and added finger-spelling to his repertoire. Success with Shirreff determined him to take another pupil, deaf-born this time, whose progress was so satisfactory that he gave a public exhibition of the attainments of his two pupils. In 1766 he began to advertise for more pupils in the *Scots Magazine*. Soon he had a flourishing little establishment on his hands. Three years later he was again writing to the *Scots Magazine*, offering to 'com-

* James Boswell mentions the visit to the Braidwood Academy in his *Tour to the Hebrides* and says that Dr Johnson asked if the pupils could pronounce any *long* words. He was told they could. 'Upon which Dr Johnson wrote one of his *sesquipedalia verba*, which was pronounced by the pupils, and he was satisfied.'

municate his skill to three or four ingenious young men who may assist and succeed him in this business' on condition that 'some kind of fund be established ... for defraying the expense of educating such'. Braidwood pointed out that 'in an age distinguished by so many public charities and so ready to encourage every invention in arts or science, a fund sufficient for the purpose might be obtained' and was not above concluding with a hint of moral blackmail: 'If Mr Braidwood receives no public encouragement, he will be obliged to move in the same confined task as hitherto, and teach only deaf persons who can afford the expense; and when he dies his valuable gift will probably die with him.'

No public encouragement, at least in terms of cash, was then forthcoming. None the less Braidwood's school continued to flourish, since its pupils were drawn from well-to-do families. In due course Braidwood felt the time had come to emigrate to greener pastures in the south. In 1783 he shifted his establishment to Hackney in London. He brought in two nephews, John Braidwood (who married one of his daughters) and Joseph Watson, thus establishing the Braidwood succession. But before pursuing the history of this family, it is necessary to take a look at what had been happening in Europe in the meantime.

The pattern of development on the Continent was similar to that in Britain. There were the intellectuals whose speculations on the nature of language led to their involvement with the practical question of teaching deaf mutes to speak; then there were the early professionals who made a livelihood from their skill as teachers of the deaf. Of the first group the outstanding names are those of Francis Mercurius, Baron Helmont (1618-99), a Belgian chemist and occultist, son of the more famous chemist who invented the word 'gas'; and John Conrad Amman (1668-1730), a Swiss physician who emigrated to the Netherlands. Like their British contemporaries Bulwer, Wallis, and Dalgarno, they were fascinated by the problem of language. However, the two continentals were mainly interested in its mystical origin. Thus Helmont put forward the theory that Hebrew was the 'natural' language of man, and published a curious book to show that the shape and character of each letter of the Hebrew alphabet conformed to the position of the organs of speech when making the sound.* Helmont made useful observations on lipreading, while

* As will be seen, in the nineteenth century Alexander Melville Bell,

his friend Amman, who was more interested in teaching articulation than language, published a book called *Surdus Loquens* (The Talking Deaf Man) in 1692, after successfully instructing a Dutch girl, Esther Collard. It was the fullest and most valuable description of techniques of teaching deaf mutes speech and lip-reading since Bonet's treatise, and proved equally influential. Thanks to the interest taken by Dr John Wallis, with whom Amman corresponded, it was published in an English translation only two years later. In 1700 he followed it up with his *Dissertatio de loquela*. These two books, with their insistence on the importance of speech, became the foundation stone of what was later to be known as the 'German system' or oral method of teaching the deaf.

Of the professional teachers of the deaf in Europe the most brilliant was a refugee Spanish Jew, Jacob Rodríguez Pereira, who was born in 1715 and is said to have begun by teaching his sister, who was deaf and dumb, to speak. Pereira's family settled at Bordeaux, where the young man began to make a name for himself as a teacher of the deaf. In 1745 he undertook the instruction of a sixteen-year-old deaf-mute aristocrat. He succeeded so admirably that in 1749 the French Academy of Sciences set up a commission of inquiry under the famous naturalist the Comte de Buffon to report on Pereira's achievement. As a result the Duc de Chaulmes presented Pereira to Louis XV. Soon Pereira was teaching the duke's deaf-born godson, Saboureaux de Fontenay. His education proved to be Pereira's masterwork. The boy achieved a higher degree of culture and learning than any deaf-born person before him – he even learned a second language – though his teacher was honest enough to note that his deafness was 'of the second degree'. But like his British contemporaries Henry Baker and Thomas Braidwood, Pereira depended on his teaching for a livelihood, and regarded his techniques as professional capital. He would not publish his method, wishing to keep it 'a secret which ought to be perpetuated by my family alone'. It is known

---

father of the inventor of the telephone, went one better and in his book *Principles of Visible Speech* introduced an alphabet, or set of symbols, each letter of which was a diagrammatic hieroglyph of the position of the speech-organs in the act of pronouncing it. The reader had merely to place his lips, tongue, etc., in the position shown by the hieroglyph and to utter the sound it represented!

that he used his own version of the one-handed finger alphabet advocated by Bonet, and that he concentrated on speech, lipreading, and the natural development of language through conversational exercises. Pereira, who has been called 'the greatest teacher of them all', probably owed his outstanding success to a natural gift plus unending patience and ingenuity – qualities that could not be transmitted by a published method, or handed down to those who did not naturally possess them (Pereira's son and widow tried, but failed, to carry on his school). He died in 1780, famous and honoured, having been made a Fellow of the Royal Society and rewarded with a pension by the king of France.

We now come to one who is far and away the greatest figure in the history of the education of the deaf, whose work was to have a profound influence on their welfare and whose educational method was to split their teachers into two camps for a century and more. He was slightly older than Pereira and Braidwood: an obscure French priest who did not begin his teaching career until he was nearly fifty. The Abbé Charles Michel de l'Épée was born in 1712 at Versailles, the son of an architect in the royal service. For a quarter of a century the Abbé remained a humble cleric: his Jansenist leanings stood in the way of advancement. In 1750 chance took him to a house where two young girls were living. When the Abbé spoke to them, they did not answer; their mother explained that they could neither hear nor speak. The encounter was a great shock to the priest. 'Believing that the two children would live and die in ignorance of their religion if I did not attempt some means of instruction, I was touched with compassion, and told the mother she might send them daily to my house, and that I would do whatever I might find possible for them,' he wrote long afterwards. As with Ponce de León, the Abbé's motive in teaching the deaf was religious.

De l'Épée taught the two sisters to read and write, and soon began to take on other pupils. At first he improvised his own techniques, till one day he was offered a copy of Bonet's famous treatise. The Abbé was about to turn it down because he knew no Spanish when he caught sight of the engraving of the one-hand alphabet that illustrated the work. He bought the book on the spot and began learning Spanish in order to read it. Next he got hold of Amman's *Dissertatio de loquela*. These two books, he afterwards wrote, were 'two torches which lighted me on my way, but in the application of their principles I have followed the route which appeared to me to be easiest and quickest'. Unlike his predecessors, de l'Épée was not content with teaching a few select deaf mutes to read, write, and articulate. He felt it imperative to give *all* who were deaf, whether rich or poor, bright or dull, a means whereby they could think, communicate, understand; and above all receive the religious instruction that he believed to be necessary for the salvation of their souls.

How was this to be done? Teaching articulate language was a long, laborious process for both teacher and pupil, each pupil requiring so much individual attention and coaching that only a few at a time could be successfully taught by a single instructor. Besides, teaching articulation took up time that could be better spent giving the pupil an education in depth. Some quicker and easier mode of communication, some simpler vehicle of thought and reason must be found.

As a young man de l'Épée had speculated about the symbolic nature of language. He may have been struck by Socrates' remark in the *Cratylus* of Plato:

If we had neither voice nor tongue, and yet wished to manifest things to one another, should we not, like those which are at present mute, endeavour to signify our meaning by the hands, head, and other parts of our body? ... I think, therefore, that if we wished to signify that which is upwards and light, we should raise our hands towards the heaven, imitating the nature of the thing itself; but that if we wished to indicate things downwards and heavy, we should point with our hands to the earth ...

De l'Épée carefully observed and studied the signs and gestures by which his pupils communicated with one another. It did not take him long to convince himself that gestures and signs were the natural language or 'mother-tongue' of the deaf-born, and that it could be the basis of a visual language wherein signals took the place of vocables. He therefore set out to construct and codify a sign language based on the 'natural signs' that he had learnt from his own pupils. This sign language was not another finger alphabet for spelling out words: each sign, rather like a Chinese ideograph, represented a word or phrase instead of a letter or phonetic element. De l'Épée evolved a combination of mime and arbitrary signs, obeying grammatical laws, systematized into a visual equivalent of spoken language. Nouns and verbs were mimed – gestured ideographs as it were – while grammatical inflections and parts of speech like prepositions and the definite article were shown by arbitrary or invented gestures. These he called *signes méthodiques*. For example he systematized a gesture used by his pupils to indicate that some action or happening was in the past (a backwards flick of the hand over the shoulder) to give the past tense of verbs. Thus one flick of the hand stood for the simple past tense, two for the perfect and three for the pluperfect. A preposition like 'for' was shown by pressing a finger on the forehead (the head=reason or intention) then pointing it towards the object. It was, in fact, a true language, independent of speech and hearing, dependent instead on the hand and eye. Complicated as it seems when described, de l'Épée's sign language – a much-modified form of which is still used in America and elsewhere – can be 'spoken' and understood with unbelievable rapidity by adepts. Those who saw the film 'Johnny Belinda' may remember the deaf child saying the Lord's Prayer in sign language, and how easily comprehensible it appeared to those who had never seen it before.

De l'Épée did teach articulation, but it was given a subordinate place in his educational programme. If his pupils could not *speak* very well, they could express themselves, in writing, in correct and even elegant French. By the oral system, as de l'Épée never tired of pointing out, deaf mutes had often been taught to articulate intelligibly without really understanding the words they spoke. The great advantage of the sign language was the ease and rapidity with which it could be taught from scratch (two years or less in some cases); consequently a greater number of deaf children could be taught. In addition his sign system was in effect a universal language that could be used by all nationalities. As Hodgson remarks, 'by reason of this wholly new kind of effort to teach children in the mass, de l'Épée became the first teacher to utter a serious challenge to what had come to be the accepted idea that to teach the deaf was to teach speech. He not only maintained that speech was not essential to the education of the deaf, but even that it was not necessarily the best way of educating them.'

Thus the Abbé de l'Épée began a debate, which is not yet wholly resolved, between the 'oral' and the 'silent' systems of educating the deaf. In the Abbé's lifetime the great 'oralist' opponent of the new method was Samuel Heinicke (1729-90). This German ex-guardsman had begun his teaching career in 1754 by instructing a deaf and dumb boy at Dresden. At the outbreak of the Seven Years' War Heinicke found himself called back to the colours. The Prussians took him prisoner, but he escaped his captors. For two or three years Heinicke was on the run, finally settling down at Hamburg where he again took up teaching the deaf. He based his method squarely on the work of Amman, and prospered so well that eventually the Elector of Saxony asked him to take charge of the first school for the deaf and dumb in Germany, which opened in 1778 at Leipzig and eventually became a family monopoly. Heinicke was the father of 'pure oralism' or what is sometimes called the 'German system'. He took his stand on the fact that it is only through articulate speech that the deaf can find a place in ordinary society. The philosophy of 'pure oralism' is the exact opposite of de l'Épée's, eschewing the use of signs and gestures of any kind, including even the finger alphabet. Heinicke contended that the use of signs hinders the acquisition of speech, just as the availability of a pair of crutches may prevent a cripple from making the attempt to walk. The sole instrument of the instruction of the deaf should therefore be spoken language. In 1782 Heinicke entered upon a controversy by letter with the Abbé de l'Épée about the merits of their respective systems. This correspondence was later submitted to the judgement of the Zürich Academy, which pronounced in favour of the Abbé – largely because Heinicke was extremely cagey about his actual methods of teaching. Thus his secretiveness retarded the advance of the oral method he advocated. For while Heinicke published no full account of his teaching techniques, the Abbé was a proselytizer and lost no opportunity of publicizing his system. He published a description of it in 1776, followed in 1784 by a revised and enlarged version – *La veritable Manière d'instruire les sourds et muets, confirmée par une longue expérience.*

The Abbé may not have achieved results like Pereira's or Heinicke's with individual pupils whose intelligence and ability, helped by painstaking coaching, enabled them not only to speak but achieve a remarkable measure of intellectual progress. On the other hand he was able to give language of a sort to very many deaf children who would otherwise have led isolated lives. And it must be said that the sign language is a very flexible medium of expression. Just as in articulate speech one can modify the sense of a word by tone of voice, so the meaning of a sign can be modified (or given an ironical or pejorative sense) by an expressive variation of gesture while making it. The drawback was that the Abbé's sign language, while it enabled the deaf to talk to each other and to their teachers, was of not much use outside that little world. The oralists aimed at fitting their pupils to take a place in ordinary society, while the Abbé – who went so far as to declare that 'the language of signs is the one form in which the deaf and dumb can think' and 'the visible form of language is alone suitable for the deaf and dumb' – was intent on providing a utilitarian vehicle of communication and reason for as many as possible of those who would otherwise pass their whole existence without any at all. His charity and saintliness make his contemporaries seem venal by comparison: 'The rich only come to my house by tolerance,' he once declared. At one period he was teaching as many as sixty children, whom he also clothed and fed out of his own pocket (it is said that he set aside only one-seventh of his income for his own needs). In 1760 he founded the Institut Nationale des Sourds-Muets in Paris. Teachers from all over Europe were sent to him for training; as a result, the 'silent' system was established in many other countries, and the first state school for the deaf founded in Austria.

When, in the year of the French Revolution, the Abbé de l'Épée died, his work was carried on by the greatest of his disciples, the Abbé Sicard. Born in 1742, Sicard had been trained by de l'Épée. Later he opened a school of his own for the deaf at Bordeaux. When in 1790 the revolutionary National Assembly gave the Abbé de l'Épée's school at Paris new premises and a government grant, it was the Abbé Sicard who was chosen to be its principal. During the Terror of 1792 he was arrested as a non-conforming priest and narrowly escaped death at the hands of the mob. After a time in hiding he eventually returned to the Institute to resume his work for the deaf. The rest of his life he devoted to elaborating and classifying de l'Épée's sign language. Sicard died in 1822, four years after publishing his magnum opus, the *Théorie des signes*, a grammar and dictionary of the sign language.

Thus the eighteenth century ended with the practicability of deaf education firmly established, and with the emergence of two rival systems – the 'oral' and the 'silent' – whose advocates were to do battle in the next hundred years. The first schools, and even the first state school, had been founded. The Abbé de l'Épée's most valuable contribution had not been the invention and dissemination of his sign language, however much it lightened the burden of so many deaf lives. Though the sense of social responsibility grew as the industrial revolution developed, it was the Abbé's charitable example that did most to implant the idea that something should be done for all deaf mutes, that from now on it was no longer permissible for society to neglect and forget the prisoners of silence.

Twelve

THE middle of the eighteenth century had seen the opening of the first schools for the deaf. With the exception of the Abbé de l'Épée's they were for the lucky few – the children of parents well-off enough to pay the fees of professional teachers. But by the end of the eighteenth century the seeds of public education for the deaf and of communal responsibility for their welfare had been sown. In the next hundred years these were to grow and proliferate; not always happily. The nineteenth century was also marked by certain medical advances, by the first legislation for deaf education and welfare, by the emergence of missions for the adult deaf and the formation of such bodies as the National Association of Teachers of the Deaf and the British Deaf and Dumb Association. Then there was the rivalry, almost the war, between advocates of the oral and silent systems of teaching the deaf.

To follow the course of deaf education and welfare in Britain we must pick up the Braidwood family saga at the point where Braidwood moved his famous Academy from Edinburgh to London in 1783, and with his two nephews set up a new school at Hackney. These nephews, Joseph Watson and John Braidwood,* were trained in his methods by Thomas Braidwood, but sworn to secrecy. At this time and for long after the family had virtually the monopoly of teaching the deaf in Britain. Thus when in 1792 a charitable scheme was mooted for the establishment of a school for the deaf children of the poor, it was natural, even inevitable, that one of the Braidwoods should become its first principal. In any case the idea came from the mother of one of Braidwood's pupils, who roped in the Rev. John Townsend, a well-known Congregational minister, the Rev. Henry Cox Mason, Rector of Bermondsey, and the philanthropist Henry Thornton to found the Asylum for the Support and Education of the Deaf and

---

* He married Thomas Braidwood's daughter and died young in 1798, but left his widow and two sons, John and Thomas, to carry on the family connexion.

Dumb Children of the Poor. This was the beginning of the 'asylum system'. Such schools, or asylums as they generally and often only too accurately called themselves, were supported by public charity and run by committees who appointed their principals or superintendents. The state had no hand in their financing (not till 1832 was the principle of state aid for education established in Britain). The London Asylum at Bermondsey opened in November 1792 with six children of either sex. Amazingly enough, the committee had doubted whether enough pupils would be found to justify the school. Four years later there were twenty and a waiting list of fifty. When in 1809 the Asylum moved to roomier quarters in the Old Kent Road the numbers had quadrupled. There the teaching of various trades was introduced, and by 1820 some two hundred deaf children were being looked after.

The first principal of the London Asylum was Braidwood's nephew Watson. He was paid no salary whatever: there was an odd and not very far-sighted arrangement by which he was expected to make his living from his profits on contracts for school supplies and from taking private pupils who paid fees. The result, of course, was that Watson and his successors came to concentrate on their fee-paying pupils and leave the others to the care of assistant teachers. As far as food and clothing went the children appear to have been well looked after, but only the fee-payers received proper instruction. Nevertheless Watson, like his uncle, seems to have been an excellent teacher. When old Thomas Braidwood died in 1806 Watson felt so far released from his pledge of secrecy that he published his *Instruction of the Deaf and Dumb* (1809). From this it can be seen that Braidwood's method was based on Dr Wallis's, elaborated and improved by his practical experience as a teacher. Watson was not a 'pure oralist' like Heinicke but permitted his pupils to use signs to begin with, though neither he nor the other Braidwoods had any use for the Abbé de l'Épée's methodological sign system. For thirty-seven years Watson remained superintendent at the Old Kent Road, until he died, a fairly rich man, in 1829. His son Thomas succeeded him and remained in charge of the Asylum for a further twenty-eight years. On his death in 1857, Thomas's son, the Rev. James Watson – the great-great-nephew of the original Thomas Braidwood – took over. After a reign of twenty-one years the last of the Watsons was more or less made to resign in 1878.

When he went, the Watson dynasty had ruled the Asylum at Old Kent Road for almost a century.

Unluckily neither the son nor the grandson of Joseph Watson inherited his talents, and assistants were neither well paid nor properly trained. While the children may have been adequately fed, the standard of teaching fell lower and lower. By the time of the last Watson pupils were barely being taught to speak or lip-read: teaching was carried on by means of a debased system of signs. Written exercises were faked for the benefit of investigating committees. Richard Elliott (who took over and reformed the Old Kent Road Asylum in 1878 after having been assistant master there for many years) painted a Dickensian picture of conditions under the last two Watsons. They were, alas, typical of some of the other asylum-schools for the deaf and dumb in mid-Victorian England: prison-like, overcrowded and understaffed establishments from which the children emerged at puberty almost as uncouth as when they went in, and with no discernible future but the workhouse.

The founding of the Old Kent Road Asylum had been followed eighteen years later by the establishment of the Edinburgh Institute in 1810. Its administration was in the hands of the same charitable committee that looked after the London Asylum. Not surprisingly, another Braidwood was given the post of superintendent – John Braidwood, grandson of old Thomas Braidwood. Two years later, the General Institution for the Instruction of Deaf and Dumb Children was opened at Birmingham with yet another Braidwood grandson as principal – Thomas Braidwood, the brother of John. At this time four schools for the deaf existed in the kingdom, all run by members of the Braidwood family – the Asylum at Old Kent Road under Joseph Watson, the Institutes at Edinburgh and Birmingham in the charge of his cousins, the two Braidwood brothers, while Mrs Braidwood, their widowed mother, still kept the old Braidwood Academy at Hackney. This remarkable situation was to have a decisive effect on the course of the education of the deaf in the United States of America.

John Braidwood, though brilliant as a teacher, was an alcoholic. Within two years of taking up his post he had to leave not only the Edinburgh Institute but the country, sailing to America in 1812, the year the British burnt Washington – hardly the best time to emigrate to the U.S. But Braidwood had an influential friend – William Bolling, the brother of three former deaf pupils at the old Braidwood Academy. With Bolling's help he eventually opened a school at Richmond in Virginia. Two of the pupils were Bolling's own children; for deafness ran in the family. Before the school could be established, Bolling had to bail Braidwood out of a debtor's prison in New York, where he had 'squandered in drink and debauchery the funds entrusted to him'. After this Bolling was continually coming to Braidwood's rescue and setting him up on his feet, till in 1819 Braidwood died, 'a victim of the bottle'.

John's brother Thomas had a better record at Birmingham but does not seem to have been as gifted a teacher. He held his post until his death in 1825. This marked the end of sixty years of Braidwood domination of the teaching of the deaf, though the Watson branch of the family was to hold out for another half-century. It also marked the end of the oral method of teaching in England for very many years. For Braidwood's successor at Birmingham, a Swiss named Louis de Puget, introduced de l'Épée's silent system.* The great commendation of the silent method of teaching, especially where schools were crowded and understaffed, was that it was easier and enabled instruction to be given to larger classes. For this reason oral teaching had either been abandoned in the other asylum-schools of Britain, or was by then merely vestigial.

Not till the early nineteenth century did the care and education of the deaf begin to get under way in America. But once fairly started the Americans moved with a pace and confident energy that left European efforts in this field standing. John Braidwood's abortive attempts to set up an oral school did not mark the true beginning of deaf education in the U.S. Had he not been an alcoholic, its history there might have been very different.

The earliest American attempt to teach the deaf may have been in 1679 when one Philip Nelson was said to have 'cured' a deaf and dumb boy called Isaac Kilbourne at Rowley, Massachusetts. The neighbours suspected witchcraft; an investigation was ordered. No one seems sure whether this was really an effort to teach a deaf mute speech. In 1773 we hear of a deaf boy called John Edge being taught in a school at Fredericksburg in Virginia. But until the nineteenth century Americans who could afford it

* According to Hodgson, there is a tradition that the pupils mutinied and demanded a return to the oral method of teaching!

sent their deaf children to Europe to be educated. A deaf nephew of President Monroe was taught at Paris, while many American pupils attended the famous Braidwood Academy at Edinburgh. Among them, in 1780, was the deaf mute son of a Bostonian called Francis Green, who was so impressed by the progress of his son and by the Academy that in 1783 he published a little book, *Vox Oculis Subjecta*,* describing the school and what he could gather of Braidwood's methods. Like Dr Johnson ten years earlier, he was particularly struck by the happiness of the school and its pupils at a time when schools were not notably happy places. In addition Francis Green made an eloquent appeal for funds to provide for the training of teachers in Braidwood's method, and for the education of the deaf children of the poor. Though the book was published in Britain, notice was taken of it in one or two American journals.† When Green returned to the U.S. he did what he could to propagate the idea of a school for the deaf in America. But he had no success, beyond instigating in 1803 a census of the deaf in New England, by which it was estimated there might be some 500 in the whole country.

A little later, around 1810, the Reverend John Stanford, a New York prison chaplain began attempting to teach deaf children he found in almshouses. This effort attracted the notice of some rich philanthropists of the city who had been interested by Green's book and by John Braidwood's stumbling attempts to set up a school for the deaf. They conducted a census of the deaf in New York (like the charitable founders of the London Asylum, they were doubtful whether there were enough deaf mutes to justify the establishment of a special school). The result was the founding of the New York Institution for the Instruction of the Deaf and Dumb (now the New York School for the Deaf) in 1818, with a roll-call of thirty-three pupils. But a year earlier, at Hartford, Connecticut, the first permanent institution for the education of the deaf in America had already opened its doors. This was the famous American Asylum. The story of its inception is characteristic of the enterprise, energetic philanthropy, public-

* 'The voice subject to the eye' – the motto of the Braidwood Academy.
† The first work on deafness to be printed in America appeared ten years later, in 1793. This was *Cadmus: A Treatise on the Elements of Written Language*, to which was appended an essay on a method of teaching articulation to the deaf. The author was a Dr Williams Thornton of Philadelphia.

spiritedness and drive that marked the first decades of the Republic.

In Hartford lived a Dr Mason Fitch Cogswell whose two-year-old daughter, Alice, lost her hearing through scarlet fever in 1807. Soon her speech began to go. Her father became anxious about her education. Since he did not want to send his daughter to Europe and no school for the deaf existed in the United States, the solution was to create one. Dr Cogswell's first step was to appeal to the local Association of Congregational Clergymen for help in taking a census of the deaf in Connecticut to establish whether there were enough deaf mutes of school age to make the enterprise feasible. Eighty-four deaf mutes were found to be living in Connecticut in 1812, and about 2,000 (it was calculated) in the whole of the U.S. Armed with these figures Dr Cogswell called a meeting in 1815 of ten of the most prominent citizens of Hartford – business men, merchants, and clergy – to put to them the general case for educating the deaf in America as well as the specific proposition to open a school at Hartford.

A decision was taken to find the money to send some suitable person to investigate European methods of teaching the deaf and dumb. The next day enough funds had been raised and the day after that a young preacher called Thomas Hopkins Gallaudet had accepted the commission; a month later he sailed for England.

Gallaudet had been born at Philadelphia in 1787 and had graduated at Yale. He was one of those present at Dr Cogswell's meeting, for recently he had come to know the doctor, and had even begun the instruction of little Alice Cogswell with the help of a book by the Abbé Sicard. Though his plans for his future career did not include teaching the deaf, Gallaudet allowed himself to be persuaded to undertake the trip to Europe.

In England he found all but one of the schools for the deaf in the hands of the Braidwood family. Old Thomas Braidwood's daughter had the Academy at Hackney, her cousin Joseph Watson the Asylum at Old Kent Road, her son Thomas the Institute at Birmingham. Even the Edinburgh school was run by one Robert Kinniburgh who was under bond to keep the family secrets. Gallaudet proposed to learn the oral method of teaching the deaf at one or other of these establishments, compare it with the French or silent system, then select what seemed to him the best elements of both. But the Braidwoods had other ideas. For one thing they were bitterly antagonistic to the French system, and for another John Braidwood was then in America trying to start an oral school for the deaf. Joseph Watson offered to send one of his assistants to America to help to establish the proposed school at Hartford. But Gallaudet thought it would be a mistake to have a teacher 'wedded to Dr Watson's mode' since he wished the projected school to combine 'the peculiar advantages of both the French and English modes of instruction'. Next Watson offered to teach Gallaudet the oral method provided he agreed to bind himself as an assistant teacher for three years, working eleven hours a day in the asylum for a nominal salary. Gallaudet declined.

At this time the Abbé Sicard, de l'Épée's successor at the Paris Institute, happened to be in London on a lecture tour. He had with him two of his deaf pupils. When Gallaudet went to see them, Sicard promptly invited him to come to Paris, where he was given a crash course in the silent system. Three months later, accompanied by one of Sicard's deaf pupil-teachers, Laurent Clerc, he sailed back to America, having been away for fifteen months.

The next thing was to raise funds to establish the school. For eight months Gallaudet and Clerc toured the principal towns and cities of America raising subscriptions and enlisting public sympathy for the cause of deaf education. Here Clerc proved invaluable as an example of what education might do for deaf mutes. He could not speak, but was able to write in French and English, thus 'exciting universal wonder and admiration'. In October 1816 the Legislature of Connecticut gave $5,000 of public money for the project – 'the first appropriation of public money made in America on behalf of a benevolent institution'* – while a further $12,000 came from private donations. In 1817 the first permanent school for the education of deaf mutes in America opened at Hartford with seven pupils, of whom Alice Cogswell was one.

By the end of the year the number had risen to thirty-three. In 1819 the Congress of the United States, under a motion made by Henry Clay, gave the school 23,000 acres of public land. Out of this grant buildings were erected to house the school and a permanent fund established. The State of Massachusetts, in that

* Edward Miner Gallaudet, *Life of Thomas Hopkins Gallaudet* (New York, 1888).

same year, made provision for twenty deaf children to be sent to the American Asylum at public expense. Other states quickly followed the lead, while some began to build their own schools. Thus 'education for the deaf was established in the United States, from the beginning, as a public responsibility'.*

From that time America led the way in munificence of provision for the deaf. This was chiefly the work of Gallaudet, who became the first principal of the American Asylum at Hartford. He was responsible for the American tradition of adequate expenditure on deaf education which, as Hodgson observes, 'has amply justified itself in the high tax-assessments of many deaf graduates' – one way of looking at it. Indeed 1817, the year of the opening of the American Asylum, was a watershed in the history of the deaf. For in that year Denmark became the first country in the world to make the education of the deaf compulsory, anticipating most other European states by half a century.

Another long-term effect of Gallaudet's enterprise was the dominance of the silent system of deaf education in America. This was almost entirely due to the jealous secretiveness of the Braidwood clan,† in sharp contrast to the generous open-handedness of the disciples of de l'Épée. By 1819 articulate speech had been abandoned at Hartford, the pupils communicating by means of sign language, the one-hand alphabet, and writing. The third annual report of the Asylum referred to oral methods as meaningless 'parlour-tricks' and 'little higher than training starlings or parrots'. Not till 1845 was any instruction given in speech or lip-reading, and it was as late as 1857 before the first teacher of articulate speech was employed at an American deaf school.

Gallaudet remained principal of the American Asylum till 1830. He married one of his deaf-born pupils in 1821. His sons followed in their father's footsteps, the elder founding the first American Church for the Deaf at New York in 1859, the younger becoming first President of Gallaudet College in Washington, D.C. This establishment, named in honour of the elder Gallaudet and inaugurated in 1864, was the first institution in the world for the higher

* Ruth E. Bender, *The Conquest of Deafness.*

† Hodgson rightly suggests that the Braidwoods may have guarded an empty cupboard. Thomas Braidwood's method derived from Dr Wallis's and owed much to his individual genius as a teacher. The later Braidwoods probably 'depended on keeping alive a belief that they did in fact possess some secret skill passed on to them by him on whose laurels they were content to rest'.

education of the deaf, and still the only one with the right to confer degrees.

Meanwhile the battle between the oral and the silent systems of deaf education continued. In the early part of the century the French or silent method appeared to be advancing everywhere. It became dominant in France, America, Italy, Spain, Scandinavia, and Germany, while oral teaching in Britain, where the asylum-schools were for long mostly in the hands of the later Braidwoods and Watsons, was either degenerating or being ousted. By 1865 it was possible for a writer in the *Quarterly Journal of Science* to observe: 'The articulation of the deaf and dumb is of rare occurrence in this country.' Yet by the end of the century it was the oralists who emerged victorious, having inflicted a shattering if not conclusive defeat upon the upholders of manual methods. This took place at the famous Conference of Teachers of the Deaf at Milan in 1880.

As we have seen, the father of 'pure oralism' was de l'Épée's German contemporary Heinicke, 'the first who proclaimed the possibility of educating deaf mutes as nature teaches the hearing'.* After Heinicke's death in 1790 the Napoleonic wars swept Europe: the Abbé de l'Épée's system came to Germany more or less in the baggage-train of the French armies. But when Napoleon fell there was a reaction against everything French. One or two German teachers began to revive the old techniques of oral teaching.

First among them was Johann Baptist Graeser (1766–1841) who never admitted the new French silent method, though it was not till the resurgence of German nationalism after Waterloo that anyone would listen to him. He was then fifty-five. Like Heinicke he believed that the only way of restoring the deaf mute to society was to give him the power of conversing like a hearing person. In 1821 Graeser made the bold experiment of attaching a deaf class to an ordinary school at Bayreuth. The idea was to give the deaf pupils a year or two of special teaching before letting them take their places in ordinary classes along with hearing children. This broke the isolation of deaf children from their hearing contemporaries, one of the worst features of even the best deaf schools. Ambitious and unorthodox as Graeser's experiment was, many of the German states took up the idea and made classes for

* Thomas Arnold, *Education of Deaf Mutes* (London, 1888).

deaf children part of the school system. Unfortunately it was a failure: the slower rate at which deaf children learn had not been sufficiently allowed for.

Another influential German adherent of oral teaching, Victor August Jager, who published an attack on sign language and finger-spelling and opposed the system of segregating the deaf, strongly advocated the idea of educating them in a normal environment. But the most seminal of German 'oralists' was Friedrich Moritz Hill. Born in 1805, he trained as a teacher under Pestalozzi, the Swiss educational reformer who had rediscovered the principles of Comenius – particularly the 'mother-method' of acquiring knowledge. This method Hill adapted for deaf children, whose speech and language he strove to develop naturally by daily use and through conversation lessons. 'Everything, everything,' he wrote, 'can be used for the teaching of language.' Hill even refused to teach writing until the child could master speech. He did not forbid the use of natural gestures in the early stages of teaching, but set his face against sign language. He trained teachers as well as publishing a great number of influential books on the education of the deaf. When he died in 1874 his disciples were everywhere.

The spread of Hill's influence was largely due to the work of one of these – David Hirsch (1813–96), for thirty-five years director of the Rotterdam School for the Deaf. Hirsch, who took most of his ideas from Hill and Jager, was a firm believer in oral techniques and even converted adherents of the silent system – most notably the Abba Balestre (1834–86). This priest visited Hirsch in 1861 and on his return to Italy spread the doctrines of oral teaching. His most important convert was the Abba Giulo Tarra (1832–89), the principal of the deaf school at Milan. Twenty years after the Abba Balestre's visit to Hirsch, the Abba Tarra was to preside over the International Congress of Teachers of the Deaf at Milan which resulted in the triumph of the oral method.

The 1860s were crucial years for the revival of oral teaching. So prevalent was the silent system by the middle of the nineteenth century, and so rapid the renaissance of the oral method, that today it is often thought that the earliest mode of instructing the deaf was the silent one. Yet, as we know, oral instruction and the teaching of speech, far from being another example of nineteenth-century progressiveness, was in fact the system practised by Ponce de León in the sixteenth century and by all his successors up to the Abbé de l'Épée, whose sign method almost completely overlaid the older tradition. Having been kept alive in Germany by teachers like Heinicke, Graeser, and Hill, the oral method became known as the 'German' system and most people supposed it to have been invented by them.* Its vigorous renaissance in Britain and America began in the 1860s. In Britain a key part in this revival was played by two of David Hirsch's trainees.

These young men, Gerrit van Asch and William van Praagh, came to England early in the decade, van Praagh at the invitation of the Baroness Mayer de Rothschild, whose husband financed Disraeli's purchase of the Suez Canal. The Baroness was anxious to have an oral teacher for her school for deaf Jewish children at Whitechapel. Van Praagh did so well that the Baroness 'determined to extend the benefits of the oral system to the afflicted of every race and creed'. She therefore used her considerable influence to found in 1872 the Association for the Oral Instruction of the Deaf and Dumb of which van Praagh became the principal. The Association opened the first training college for teachers of the deaf in Britain. Before this, hardly any teachers in British deaf schools had received any training whatever.† A few years later a very similar body was established by St John Ackers, a barrister and Member of Parliament. After an extensive tour of deaf schools in Europe and the United States, undertaken for the sake of his deaf daughter, he had been convinced by the superiority of the oral method of education. In 1877 St John Ackers founded the Society for Training Teachers of the Deaf and the Diffusion of the German Method, and in the following year the Society opened its own training college at Ealing.

This was the year that saw the end of the Watson dynasty at the Old Kent Road Asylum. Richard Elliott, the Rev. James Watson's reforming and dissatisfied former assistant, had recently become principal of the Margate Asylum, an offshoot of the London Asylum at Old Kent Road. Here Elliott began to reintroduce the teaching of speech. Next he set about organizing a conference of principals of schools for the deaf so that the superintendents of institutes and asylums could meet such progressive oral

* During the 1914–18 War some advocates of the silent method went so far as to claim that oral teaching, being German, was unpatriotic!

† At this date in Germany teachers of the deaf had to spend three years in training college, followed by two years' apprenticeship at a deaf school before becoming fully qualified: the whole paid for by the state.

teachers as van Asch, van Praagh, and Miss Susannah Hull, who in 1862 had opened a small private school in Kensington. Elliott prepared for the conference by making a tour of the various charitable asylums and institutions for the deaf that had sprung up since the founding of the London and Birmingham asylums at the turn of the century.

By 1829 charitable institutions for the deaf and dumb had opened at Glasgow, Aberdeen, and Dublin. One had been established at Manchester in 1825, and Liverpool followed suit. Yorkshire provided for some of its deaf children with a day-school at Doncaster, established in 1829 under a young man called Charles Baker, who remained its principal for forty-four years. All these places used the silent or manual system: Baker dismissed articulate speech as 'a specious accomplishment'. Many of them were dreary buildings where the inmates were isolated from the world not only by their deafness but by the asylum walls. Their bread was the bitter bread of charity. As D. G. Pritchard remarks in his *Education and the Handicapped*: 'It was this lack of contact with normality, this almost complete segregation from ordinary life, that was one of the worst features of the education of the handicapped in the first seventy years of the nineteenth century.' However, at Donaldson's Hospital at Edinburgh, which opened in 1850, destitute deaf and hearing children were accommodated together, though taught separately. The remarkably forward-looking system was a success, and lasted till 1938.

But few principals of the institutes and asylums that Richard Elliott visited welcomed new ideas. At Doncaster the new principal, James Howard, was teaching speech to a few pupils. Howard helped Elliott to organize the conference of principals of schools for the deaf which was held at London in 1877. Experts in the oral method talked to them, and they were persuaded to visit an oral school to see what skilled teaching could achieve. Nothing immediate happened – but in the next year, 1878, the Rev. James Watson resigned from the London Asylum in Old Kent Road, and Elliott was appointed in his stead. The night may not have been over, but the east was lightening.

In the meantime, an unregarded nonconformist clergyman at Northampton had quietly been making himself one of the leading practitioners of pure oralism in the country. The Rev. Thomas Arnold had already started his 'middle-class school for the deaf and dumb'. He was an Ulsterman whose forebears had come over with William of Orange. They were Moravians – an evangelical Protestant sect who at one time followed the curious practice of marriage by lot. Arnold was born in 1816 at Gracehill in Co. Antrim, the son of a cabinet-maker. When he was a boy one of the deaf-mute pupils of the Claremont Institute near Dublin came to lodge with the Arnold family in order to learn carpentry. This lad taught Arnold finger-spelling that they might talk together. But his limited vocabulary and gropings to express himself made a crucial impression on Arnold. 'I felt for him, for he uttered strange noises on these occasions. . . . This led me to endeavour to aid him,' he wrote long afterwards in an autobiographical sketch. Arnold began his career as a teacher of the deaf by joining the staff of the Manchester City Mission. This was one of the many religious-charitable welfare missions for the adult deaf that came into being during the first half of the nineteenth century. Then in 1840 Arnold became an assistant teacher in the Yorkshire Institution at Doncaster under Charles Baker. There, as in all institutions for the deaf at that time, communication was by signs and finger-spelling. 'It seemed like being among a people who spoke another language, lived a different kind of life, thought and felt unlike ourselves. . . . The sign method made them strangers, and their teachers had to become like them to understand them.' He left Doncaster for Liverpool, where some oral teaching was being given under the headmastership of James Rhind. Here Arnold taught a boy called George Cockin to speak. His experiences at Doncaster and Liverpool convinced Arnold not only that oral teaching was best for the deaf, but that any form of sign communication was incompatible with it. In 1842 Arnold was offered the headship of a new Asylum at Brighton. But when he discovered that it involved – as most posts of this sort did at the time – subscribing to the thirty-nine articles of the Anglican communion, his stubborn nonconformism would have none of it and he turned down the offer. He abandoned the teaching of the deaf, became a Congregationalist minister, married, and in 1858 emigrated to Australia.

Instead of being the end of the story, this proved a beginning. A member of the legislative council of New South Wales, the Hon. Thomas Holt, begged Arnold to educate his deaf son. Arnold accepted the task. Unluckily bad health forced his return to England after a year or two in Australia. Rather than abandon the boy's education Arnold brought young Frederick Holt back with him. In England Arnold settled down as minister of a Congregational church at Northampton, where in 1868 he was asked to take on another pupil, a seven-year-old boy from Leeds called Abraham Farrar.

The little boy was a deaf mute, having lost his hearing through scarlet fever at the age of three. For Arnold he represented an opportunity to make a crucial test of the oral method of education. Farrar achieved the breakthrough: he became the first pupil from a deaf school to pass a public examination in England. In 1881, after thirteen years with Arnold, Farrar matriculated, entered the University of London at the age of twenty, and in due course qualified as an architect and surveyor. It was a resounding achievement. Arnold regarded Farrar as convincing proof of the superiority of the oral method and of the feasibility of the higher education of the deaf. The rest of his life he devoted to these two causes.

The school at Northampton gradually expanded, though there were never more than twenty or so pupils at any one time. Arnold took on an assistant, Walter Bessant, whom he trained, and later H. N. Dixon, who succeeded as headmaster when Arnold retired from active teaching in 1884. Dixon remained until 1909. In that year Frederick Ince-Jones, who had been Dixon's assistant since 1901, became headmaster and proprietor till the school closed for good on his retirement in 1944. By a coincidence it was the same year that Abraham Farrar, the school's first and most famous pupil, died at the age of eighty-three. It was under Ince-Jones that this little school reached its apogee with a consistent and unparalleled record of public-examination successes. For eighty years Arnold's school remained the only institution in Britain for the higher education of the deaf.

Apart from his practical teaching Arnold wrote many books, including *Education of Deaf Mutes: A Manual for Teachers* (1888) which is still a standard text-book and the Bible of the oral method – the last edition appeared in 1954. The revising and rewriting of this book occupied Abraham Farrar for much of his life. It was written by Arnold specifically for the College of the Teachers of the Deaf, which he helped to form in 1885.

Thus from the 1860s onward the oral teaching of the deaf began to gain ground everywhere. Even in France and America, the strongholds of the silent systems, it found adherents and converts. In France Jean-Jacques Valade-Gabel, a teacher at the Paris Institute for Deaf Mutes from 1825 to 1838, was like Hill a student of Pestalozzi. Eventually he became Inspector-General of Institutions for the Deaf in France, and did what he could to promote the Pestalozzi system of teaching language by use. This paved the way for the eventual adoption of oral techniques by the French schools for the deaf.

In America well-appointed residential schools – in complete contrast to the miserable asylums and institutes in Britain – had sprung up everywhere, though all followed the silent system, finger-spelling and signs. However the educationalist Horace Mann (1796–1859), who had advocated the state school system in America, began to interest himself in the education of the handicapped. He joined forces with Dr Samuel Gridley Howe (1808–76), principal of the Massachusetts School for the Blind.* The two men toured European schools for the deaf in 1843, returning enthusiastic converts to the oral method. Horace Mann published a report advocating its use in America, which attracted some attention from the parents of deaf children. But other American teachers of the deaf who visited Europe were far less impressed and saw no reason to change from the silent system. When a group of parents, backed by Dr Howe, petitioned in 1864 for an oral school for the deaf to be established in Massachusetts by the state, the petition was turned down because expert witnesses from the American Asylum at Hartford favoured the silent method introduced by Gallaudet. This preference arose from the emphasis placed by American educationalists on the economic survival of the deaf after leaving school. In American state schools for the deaf priority was given to vocational training, for which they were well and sometimes lavishly equipped. As Hodgson says, the Americans saw that

a thorough training for the business of life was, in the long view, the cheapest policy. It meant deaf people paying taxes and adding to the

---

* Dr Howe was famous as the first teacher of the deaf and blind girl Laura Bridgman, an achievement celebrated by Charles Dickens in his *American Notes* (1842). Howe taught her language by means of raised print and the finger alphabet, and later wished he had tried to teach her to speak. When Hellen Keller lost sight and hearing in infancy her mother remembered Dickens's graphic account of the education of Laura Bridgman and was inspired to find a teacher for her daughter – with results we all know.

national income, instead of a horde of people who, having been a great expense throughout their schooldays, remain a great expense for the rest of their lives because they cannot remain in employment. They saw, as the English never saw, that in education to be penny wise is in the long run to be pound foolish.

Looked at from this angle the oral method could be said to be unrealistic not only because it was slow and difficult but because it concentrated on producing pupils who could speak and not enough on the problem of equipping them to earn a living in competition with the hearing.

On the other hand well-off American parents who could provide for their deaf children were less worried about their ability to earn a living than that they should be capable of entering normal society. From this point of view speech and lipreading were all-important. A group of such parents, led by Senator Gardiner Hubbard, whose daughter had lost her hearing at the age of four, determined to have oral instruction for their children. As a result a small private school for teaching the deaf speech was established in 1867 at Chelmsford, Massachusetts, under Harriet Rogers, whose sister had been one of Laura Bridgman's teachers. Meanwhile Senator Hubbard again petitioned the Governor of Massachusetts for an oral school. His letter coincided on the Governor's desk with another, written by a wealthy banker called John Clarke, containing an offer of $50,000 towards the founding of an oral school for the deaf to be built at Northampton, Massachusetts. Members of the Massachusetts State Legislature were taken to meet Harriet Roger's pupils to see for themselves what oral teaching could achieve. They were so impressed that by October 1867 the Clarke School for the Deaf had opened its doors at Northampton, with Harriet Rogers as its first principal.

That the two most famous oral schools for the deaf in the English-speaking world should have been founded at almost the same time in towns of the same name is an almost Joycean coincidence. Like its British namesake the American school at Northampton became a cradle of the revival of the oral method. In its first three years it received donations totalling $300,000, while similar schools, notably the Horace Mann School at Boston* and the New York Institution for the Improved Instruction of Deaf Mutes, were established.

* Helen Keller was to be its most famous pupil.

Against this background of perseverance in and development of the techniques of oral teaching the International Conference of Teachers of the Deaf convened at Milan in 1880. Over a hundred and fifty delegates from every country in the world that had schools for the deaf attended. The strong British contingent included Thomas Arnold and Richard Elliott; America sent the two sons of Thomas Hopkins Gallaudet; the Germans, French, and Italians were represented in force. On the first day the Conference elected its officers, choosing for its President the Abba Tarra, who had been converted to the teaching of speech by the Abba Balestre after the latter's visit to Hirsch's Rotterdam school for the deaf nineteen years before. The atmosphere was one of fervour and enthusiasm. The Abba Tarra delivered an inaugural address of such eloquence and fire that it brought everyone to their feet shouting 'Evviva la parola!' (Long live speech!) On the second day the Conference plunged straight into a discussion of methods of teaching the deaf. Papers were read by advocates of the silent, oral and 'combined'* systems, with Thomas Arnold of Northampton as principal champion of the pure oral method of teaching, and Dr Gallaudet, president of Gallaudet College, of the 'combined' system. Speech won the day. The following resolution was put to the meeting and carried by an overwhelming vote:

The Congress, considering the incontestable superiority of speech over signs in restoring the deaf mute to society, and in giving him a more perfect knowledge of language, declares that the oral method ought to be preferred to that of signs for the education and instruction of the deaf and dumb.

In the next few days the Congress went further, and adopted the resolution that the 'pure oral method' should be preferred 'considering that the simultaneous use of speech and signs has the disadvantage of injuring speech, lipreading, and precision of ideas'. As important, or even more important, was the resolution urging 'That Governments should take the necessary steps that all the deaf and dumb may be educated' (not till 1893 was the education of deaf children made compulsory in England). Other resolutions recommended that the schooling of deaf children should begin

* The name given to any compromise between the oral and manual methods, e.g. when the use of signs and finger-spelling is permitted in the early stages of education, or throughout. The term was first used by Dr E. M. Gallaudet in 1867. To 'pure oralists' the 'combined' systems were as much anathema as the silent.

between the ages of eight and ten (very late by modern ideas) and that classes should never exceed ten pupils (this was remarkably progressive, considering that classes of sixty were thought reasonable in hearing schools at that time).

The Conference received full publicity from newspapers: *The Times* of London reported it daily. Subsequently all countries, with the exception of the United States, adopted the oral method as the preferred system of instruction. Governments were spurred into beginning to take on the responsibility of financing and supervising the education of the deaf. In a moment of euphoria, the resolutions passed by the Conference were described by one of the English delegation as 'the deaf child's Magna Carta'. Perhaps it was not an exaggeration.

Thirteen

A RESULT of the Conference of Milan was to send home the French delegation quite converted to the oral system of teaching the deaf: in 1886 it became, by decree, the standard method of teaching in French schools. German and Dutch schools for the deaf were already oralist, as were most schools in Belgium and Italy. The silent system was retained longer in Sweden, which in 1889 made the education of the deaf compulsory. In Russia the deaf became the responsibility of a Curator who was answerable for their well-being to the sovereign; fifty schools for the deaf were in existence there by the beginning of the twentieth century, though, owing to a shortage of trained teachers, there was very little oral instruction. The Finns initiated a system by which deaf children from outlying parts of the country were boarded out with families who lived near deaf schools. But the real importance of the Conference of Milan was not so much its official recognition of the superiority of the oral method of deaf education as the stimulus it gave the delegates to put pressure on governments to concern themselves seriously with the care, education, and welfare of the deaf.*

In England, while education had been made compulsory in 1876, the law did not apply to deaf children. But after the Conference of Milan, English teachers of the deaf began to prod the government. Their efforts resulted in the Royal Commission on the Blind and Deaf, convened in 1885, which sat till 1889. (Incidentally, because of the difference of their problems neither the

* Even before Milan, schools for the deaf had begun to spring up all over the world, apart from Europe and the United States. Canada's first deaf school was established in Quebec as early as 1831, though it lasted only a few years; another was opened in 1848 at Montreal. The first institution for the deaf in Australia was opened at Sydney in 1860; Irish nuns from Cabra founded a school in South Africa three years later; while in 1879 Gerrit van Asch emigrated from England to found an oral school at Christchurch in New Zealand. The first Japanese deaf school was started in 1878, only ten years after the country had been thrown open to the West. In 1884 the first Indian school for the deaf was established in Bombay.

blind nor the deaf – or at least those working for them – were much pleased at being lumped together.) As far as the deaf were concerned the Commission did a thorough job, visiting every institution in the United Kingdom and many in France, Germany, and Italy. It found that little more than half the deaf children of Britain were being taught, and recommended compulsory education between the ages of seven and sixteen, but stepped gingerly when it came to the question of method. The advice of the Commission was that all should be given opportunity to learn to speak and lipread, but those found incapable of learning by the oral method should be taught by the manual system. However it insisted that children taught by the oral system should have no contact either in or out of school with those taught by manual methods. The Commission also recommended the development of vocational training, higher salaries for teachers of the deaf, and the establishment of an inspectorate.

Most of these recommendations were incorporated in the Elementary Education (Blind and Deaf Children) Act of 1893, which required deaf children to be educated from the age of seven to sixteen. (At this time hearing children began their schooling two years earlier; not till 1937 was the starting age for deaf children lowered to five.) A small annual grant – five guineas a head – was provided for the education and maintenance of deaf children at the institutions and asylums, the rest being found by the local rates. Local School Boards were required to build new schools where necessary. This marked the end of the old 'asylum system'. As time went on further Acts were passed, one in 1902 making some provision for the higher education of the deaf in the shape of scholarships for further training beyond the age of sixteen (which, however, were not often asked for), till in 1944 the Education Act gave legislative form to the principle that the education of deaf children 'should be an integral part of the whole educational system rather than a self-contained, self-sufficient system governed mainly by considerations not affecting other children'.*

After the Conference of Milan, America remained the fortress of the silent methods of education. But the teaching of speech and lipreading had begun to spread quickly following the establishment of the Clarke School at Northampton and the Horace Mann

* *The Education of Deaf Children* (H.M.S.O., 1968).

School at Boston in the 1860s. One of the champions of the oral method in America, and one of the great figures in the history of deafness, was Alexander Graham Bell, the inventor of the telephone. This invention, more or less a by-product of his work for the deaf, led indirectly to the development of the modern hearing-aid.

Bell came from a family of linguists and elocutionists. Both his father and grandfather (a one-time actor) were professors of elocution at Edinburgh. His father was that Alexander Melville Bell who invented 'Visible Speech' while questing (like Dr Bulwer and George Dalgarno before him) for a universal language. In his book *Principles of Visible Speech*, he introduced a more-than-phonetic alphabet each letter of which was designed to indicate the positions of the tongue and lips when uttering the sound represented by its letter or symbol. When they were boys, Alexander Melville Bell is said to have offered his sons a prize if they could make a machine able to say words – and they did produce a contraption that came near to emitting intelligible vocables.* Their mother had been deaf from an early age, yet never learned to lipread – which seems extraordinary considering the family obsession with speech and phonetics. It was in fact Bell's interest in elocution and his father's 'Visible Speech', rather than his mother's deafness, that involved him in his work for the deaf.

Alexander Graham Bell was born at Edinburgh in 1847. When he was twenty-one, soon after the death of his youngest brother from tuberculosis, the family moved to London, where young Bell met Miss Susannah Hull, who had opened a small oral school for the deaf at Kensington in 1861. With Miss Hull he began experimenting with adaptations of 'Visible Speech' for teaching her pupils articulation. It is an odd point that at this time Bell believed in speech for the deaf but not in lipreading; because his mother could not read lips he was sure it was a waste of effort. Bell had been in London for only two years when his surviving brother also died of tuberculosis and he himself was found to be infected. In the hope of saving his life the family decided to try a change of

*At Edinburgh University, appropriately enough, a machine for producing synthetic speech has recently been built by the Department of Phonetics and Linguistics. It is called a Parametric Artificial Talking Device (PAT). A similar machine is at Stockholm, and a tape exists of the two devices singing a duet: 'The More We Are Together the Merrier We Will Be.'

climate. They moved to North America in 1870 – first to Canada, then to Boston, where Bell's father was well known as a lecturer.

At Boston young Bell was snapped up by Miss Sarah Fuller, the principal of the newly opened Horace Mann oral school for the deaf, and invited to train her teachers and pupils in the use of his father's 'Visible Speech'. The results were so encouraging that after two months he went on to teach the method at the Clarke School at Northampton and at the American Asylum at Hartford. At first everyone was enthusiastic about 'Visible Speech', partly because it was new and partly because, at that time, there were no trained oral teachers of the deaf in America. It was not apparent, to begin with, how fundamentally cumbrous was a system which burdened deaf children with an extra alphabet. However, Bell opened in 1872 at Boston the first American training school for teachers of the oral method, with 'Visible Speech' as one of the techniques. (By now Bell had become a convert to lipreading, after having seen the ease with which the pupils of the Horace Mann school practised it.) The Boston training school never really got off the ground, mainly because of the opposition, or at any rate lack of support, which it encountered from the big American deaf schools. They were too firmly entrenched in the silent systems to wish for change. So Bell reverted to the family profession of teaching elocution. His training school became a 'School of Vocal Physiology'.

It will be remembered that the introduction of oral teaching of the deaf in America had been partly due to Senator Gardiner Hubbard's daughter, whose deafness had led this influential politician to play a leading role in the establishment of the Clarke School at Northampton. By 1872 Mabel Hubbard was a grown woman. She began attending Bell's elocution classes at Boston to improve her speech. Very soon the deaf girl and the young elocutionist had fallen in love. The Hubbard family were not at first enthusiastic about the match – Bell was penniless – but the Senator, who seems to have been a man of enterprise, decided to give Bell practical backing for his ideas. At that time, besides running his school of elocution, Bell had undertaken the education of George Sanders, a five-year-old deaf boy. On top of this he had begun the experiments that eventually led to the invention of the telephone. Senator Hubbard and Thomas Sanders, the grateful father of the little boy, provided the financial help Bell needed for his experiments.

When on 10 March 1876 Bell, having spilt sulphuric acid over himself, inadvertently but successfully transmitted a complete sentence over an electric wire to his assistant in the next room – 'Mr Watson, come here, I want you' – their fortunes were made. Hubbard and Sanders helped to develop the Bell Telephone Company which brought great wealth to all concerned. Bell married Mabel Hubbard in 1877.

The invention of the telephone had been the uncovenanted result of Bell's preoccupation with 'Visible Speech'. It led him, while teaching at the Horace Mann School, to experiment with the visual reproduction of speech-patterns. For this he used a manometric flame – a gas flame which pulsated according to the pressure of sound-waves. With the aid of an apparatus of revolving mirrors Bell found it possible to obtain a visual image of speech – patterns thrown by the manometric flame as it reacted to sound-waves. He thought that such a visual check might help deaf children to produce the correct sounds in speech. But the reflected patterns were too faint to be recorded photographically. As a substitute he began experimenting with the electrical transmission of sound. While doing so the basic principle of the telephone occurred to him: 'If I could make a current of electricity vary in intensity precisely as the air varies in density during the production of sound, I should be able to transmit speech telegraphically.' In the end Bell evolved a technique by which a membrane that vibrated to sound-waves at one end of a telegraph circuit induced corresponding changes in the electric current, which in turn caused identical vibrations in a membrane at the other end, thus producing the same sound-waves. The telephone was born.

Its invention was of no practical use to the deaf, but the Bell Telephone Company in the course of time spent vast sums on research in audiology which could not but benefit them. And when the French government awarded Bell the Alessandro Volta Prize of 50,000 francs for his invention, he used the money together with $100,000 of his own to found in 1887 the Volta-Bureau 'for the increase and diffusion of knowledge relating to the deaf'. Three years later Bell helped to found the American Association for Teaching Speech to the Deaf, which became a national association of teachers of the oral method. In 1908 the two bodies merged, and since 1954 they have been known as the Alexander Graham Bell Association for the Deaf. Its headquarters is the Volta Bureau, which maintains one of the world's largest libraries of books on deafness and its problems. Besides dispensing information and statistics it also published the *Volta Review*, one of the leading periodicals of the deaf world.

Bell went on to other inventions, but never lost interest in the deaf. A militant oralist, he opposed the use of sign language, though not of finger-spelling, which he regarded as a form of writing. With Bell's prestige and resources thrown into the balance, the scales were weighted in favour of oral methods of teaching the deaf in America. The turning-point probably came in 1892 when a conference of principals of deaf schools held at Colorado passed a resolution 'that in all schools for the deaf, pupils who are able to articulate ... should be encouraged to use their vocal organs on every possible occasion'. Thirty years later, at the time of Bell's death in 1922, oral methods of teaching the deaf predominated in the United States. For by 1921, according to statistics given in *American Annals of the Deaf*,* of the 14,466 pupils at the 158 deaf schools in America, 11,714 were being taught speech. Of these 10,450 were taught 'wholly or chiefly by the oral method'.

During the nineteenth century progress in the fields of science, technology, and medicine had begun to accelerate spectacularly; it was to advance even faster in the twentieth, enabling the problems of deafness to be tackled from many angles. One important result of Bell's work on the telephone was the beginning of the science of electro-acoustics, which led to the development of the modern hearing-aid after Edison (himself a deaf man) had discovered the principle of electric amplification of sound. Naturally the electric hearing-aid, as well as the audiometer (an instrument for measuring the precise degree and type of hearing loss) was to have a profound effect on the technique of deaf education. The first electric hearing-device appeared in 1900. It was a 'micro-telephone' designed and produced by Dr Ferdinand Alt of the Politzer Clinic in Vienna.

Hearing-aids have a long history, if the term admits such early

*A periodical begun by teachers at the American Asylum at Hartford and now published by Gallaudet College. This learned journal, which has appeared with only two interruptions since 1847 (one of them due to the American Civil War), constitutes a unique, almost encyclopedic historical record of everything to do with deafness and deaf education.

bugging devices as the Dome of Dionysius, a sound-amplifying domed ceiling ending in a tube that led to some other room – from a dungeon to the jailer's office, for example, or from a council-chamber to another part of the building. Huge bronze horns were used as loud-hailers by the ancients, and both Homer and Josephus refer to them. Nearer our own day there was Octacoustion, which Samuel Pepys inspected at a meeting of the Royal Society in 1668:

Here, to my great delight, I did try the use of the Otacoustion, which was only a great glass bottle broke at the bottom, putting the neck to my eare, and there I did plainly heare the dancing of the oares of the boats in the Thames ...

But the first hearing-aids designed specifically for the deaf do not seem to have appeared before the seventeenth century, when artificial horns of metal replaced animal horns that had been used up till then. In the eighteenth century the resonator trumpet, which gave much greater amplification, was introduced, and ear-trumpets of one kind or another became commonplace. Mechanical hearing-aids proliferated with truly gorgeous abandon in the next century, which was the great age of speaking-tubes, artificial ear-drums, dentaphones, acoustic chairs (a king of Portugal went so far as to commission an acoustic throne), acoustic opera-combs, acoustic top-hats, walking-sticks, and even 'beard-receptors', a sort of ear-trumpet designed to be hidden beneath one's whiskers. Collections of these fantasies may be seen at the Amplivox Hearing Centre in London, and in the Library of the Central Institute for the Deaf in America at St Louis.

Though some of these devices were capable of magnifying sound by as much as two bels, the electronic hearing-aids of the twentieth century have of course done much better. The early electronic amplifiers were cumbersome and not always efficient. It was not till 1923 that the Marconi Company put on the market the first 'portable' amplifier, the Otophone. In 1932 the first hearing-aids with miniature valves made their appearance, and in 1954 the transistor made possible the development of aids weighing only a few ounces, which could be worn by quite small children. The value of such devices in enabling those children who are not totally deaf to pick up language in the natural way, by ear, need hardly be emphasized. Apart from individual hearing-aids there are more powerful group-aids that are used in classrooms and make possible discussion and general conversation, as well as being invaluable in speech training.

Between them the audiometer and the electronic hearing-aid revolutionized the teaching of the deaf, making possible its newest development – auditory training – and the approach that is now known as audiology. These techniques were intensively explored in the thirties and forties by the Department of Education of the Deaf at Manchester University, under Irene and Alexander Ewing.

Almost since its inception in 1919 this Department has been a powerhouse for ideas, educational techniques, and research into the problems of deafness. It was endowed as a memorial to the deaf-born son of a wealthy Lancashire cotton-merchant. This brilliant young man, Ellis Llwyd Jones, had been educated so successfully by Miss Susannah Hull – the same Susannah Hull who first interested Alexander Graham Bell in teaching the deaf – that he entered the University of Oxford, thus becoming its first deaf-born undergraduate. Two years after his untimely death in 1917 his father, Sir James E. Jones, gave Manchester University £16,000 to endow 'a Department for the advancement of the Teaching of the Deaf in connexion with which the Ellis Llwyd Jones Professorship or Lectureship shall be held'. Manchester, which in 1899 had been the first English university to establish a Chair of Education, became – and remained until quite recently – the only English university with a department that deals with the education of the deaf.*

At the time of its founding the need for such a department, where teachers of the deaf might be trained, was urgent. The Royal Commission of 1889 had noted: 'The great want in the whole subject of the education of the deaf is the want of competent teachers'. Forty years later, of the two private training colleges for teachers of the deaf that were in existence at the time of the Commission, one had closed. Only the National College of Teachers of the Deaf constituted in 1918 from the old National Association of Teachers of the Deaf and the College of Teachers of the Deaf and Dumb (which the Rev. Thomas Arnold helped to found in 1885), had the right to examine teachers and confer diplomas until the department at Manchester came into existence.

When it opened in 1919 the department was modest enough,

* Similar departments have been set up in the past few years by the universities of Oxford, London, and Edinburgh.

consisting of a single room at the top floor of one of the buildings, with six students and a staff of one. Very much a pioneering venture from the beginning, it owed everything to the brilliant (but at first unpopular) choice of Miss Irene Goldsack as its first lecturer and head of department. Since 1912 Miss Goldsack had been in charge of what was in effect an experimental unit – the Henry Worral Branch of the Royal Schools for the Deaf at Manchester. This was the first residential school for young deaf children (pupils entered at five) to be opened in Britain.* As its first principal Miss Goldsack had been given carte blanche to develop and use her own methods. In contrast to the pronunciation drill based on a limited range of arbitrarily chosen words and phrases that most teachers of the deaf at that time used for teaching beginners to articulate, she had led her pupils to accept lipreading and speech by linking them with their everyday interests and activities. She had encouraged spontaneity and initiative in talking and doing, and made every effort to enlarge the children's experience of people and things. Parents were invited to come to the school and take part in the children's activities. In her last year there she had begun to experiment in making use of whatever residual hearing she could find in her pupils to help their speech and language. These were the seeds of the main developments Irene Goldsack was to foster at Manchester over the next thirty years: the earliest possible beginning of the teaching of deaf children; play-techniques; parent guidance; and auditory training.

Though one of the most important aspects of the work of the department was, and still is, the practical training of teachers of the deaf, its real contribution has lain in the development of the techniques made possible by twentieth-century advances in electronics and technology. In 1922 Miss Goldsack married Professor (later Sir Alexander) Ewing, who in 1944 was to succeed her as head of department. Together the Ewings formed a dynamic team and under them the department grew rapidly in status and achievement.

When in 1928 the department purchased a pure-tone audiometer – designed in the Bell Telephone Laboratories at New York and the first to be installed in Britain – Professor Ewing began investigating the degree and type of hearing loss among children

* The first-ever nursery school for deaf infants opened at Manchester in 1860 but had to close in 1884 because the space was needed for older children.

at deaf schools with the new instrument. Serious research into grades of deafness had not begun till as late as 1890, when a Dr James Kerr Love was appointed honorary aurist to the Glasgow Institution for the Deaf. Dr Love made the discovery that total deafness is a comparatively rare phenomenon. Less than ten per cent of the children he examined were in this class, while twenty-five per cent could hear loud speech. He advocated the classification of pupils in schools according to the severity of their deafness. As a result the first separate school for the partially deaf was opened in Scotland in 1908, though it was not till 1938 that a Departmental Committee of the Board of Education recommended that partially deaf pupils should be educated separately from the severely deaf. This was largely due to Professor Ewing's pilot investigations with the pure-tone audiometer, which confirmed and amplified Dr Love's findings and established that 'scientifically speaking, few children are totally deaf'.

In 1931 Dr T. S. Littler joined the department as its expert in electro-acoustics. He began designing improved electronic 'group-aids' and individual hearing-aids (his first model weighed 28 lb!) Even before the first serviceable hearing-aids appeared the Ewings had been using multiple speaking-tubes to harness residual hearing in order to help the speech and lipreading of deaf children and make them 'hearing-minded'. With the new improved aids designed by Dr Littler they began research into the capacity of deaf children to benefit from their use, and evolved a technique of training pupils to combine listening with lipreading. It was found that children with little residual hearing, after being trained to use these aids, learned to follow speech more accurately, to modulate their voices better and to talk more spontaneously: at the same time their progress in learning language and in general education showed improvement. These techniques and results, together with information about audiometry and hearing-aids, were described in *The Handicap of Deafness*, published by the Ewings in 1938. It was one of the first of their many books, and the first English text-book on audiology, as the new science was beginning to be called.

By the outbreak of the Second World War the Department had become an international centre for the training of teachers of the deaf and for research into all problems connected with deafness. After the war the Department was renamed 'the Department of Audiology and Deaf Education' and now conducts a post-graduate course leading to the Diploma in Audiology. Since the death of Lady Ewing and the retirement of Sir Alexander it has been headed by Professor I. G. Taylor, with Dr T. J. Watson as Reader in Deaf Education and a staff of twenty-six lecturers and research associates. The department now occupies several floors of one of the modern buildings at Manchester University, with well-equipped laboratories, clinics, and workshops.

Of the research work at Manchester the most interesting and potentially valuable has been the experimental work with very young children, involving the early detection of deafness, the assessment of intelligence of young deaf children, the evolution of parent guidance clinics, and the techniques of auditory training, which may now begin with infants of six months or even younger.* In 1948 Irene Ewing, who had been experimenting in home training for two deaf children under twelve months, and a few others aged between one and two years old, established that a twelve-month-old totally deaf baby had begun to understand speech by lipreading. Later it was found possible to fit the youngest babies with hearing-aids. Nowadays the importance and value of auditory training from the earliest possible moment is widely recognized. Basically, auditory training consists of training the residual hearing by exercising it as much as possible. As soon as the child's deafness is detected the child is made to wear an aid continuously. The parents, by talking to him as they would a hearing child, help him to pick up language and speech – or at least to make a beginning – much earlier and more naturally than would otherwise be possible. They should also help and correct his articulation, encourage him to listen to radio and television programmes – do everything, in fact, to increase and maintain his child's auditory perception and knowledge of language. The child's actual hearing will not be improved; but he can be taught to extract the utmost from what hearing he has left, with results that can be quite remarkable. According to Freddy Bloom, who describes her experience of the method in *Our Deaf Children*,† 'more and more children who were originally classified as severely or even profoundly deaf eventually learn to use a telephone ... Without auditory training those same children would have no

* One of the earliest advocates of early parental training of deaf infants was William Robson Scott (1811–77) in *The Deaf and Dumb, Their Education and Social Position.*

† Freddy Bloom, *Our Deaf Children* (1963), Heinemann.

useful hearing at all. They are just as deaf as ever they were, but they have learned the wonderful trick of using whatever hearing they have.'

The development of audiology and the results achieved by the use of audiometers and hearing-aids was one of the factors that led to the provision of separate educational arrangements for the deaf and partially deaf after the Education Acts of 1944. Special schools for partially deaf children began to be opened.* In 1962 the Handicapped Pupils and Special Schools Amending Regulations divided deaf children into two official categories, deaf and partially hearing. Interestingly enough the criterion by which a child is placed in one or other of these categories is not the severity of his hearing loss but the type of education he requires. A partially deaf child whose deafness has not been discovered till late, and who therefore has still to begin learning language and articulation, would be classified as 'deaf', while another, who may be stone deaf but did not lose his hearing until after he had acquired speech and language (as in my own case), would be classified as 'partially hearing'. The former must first of all begin learning language and speech before ordinary education can be attempted; but the latter (defined by the Amending Regulations as a pupil 'with impaired hearing, whose development of speech and language, even if retarded, is following a normal pattern'), who requires for his education 'special arrangements or facilities though not necessarily all the educational methods used for deaf pupils', will obviously benefit from classes where the other pupils have already a command of language. It is worth noting that the official circular accompanying these Amending Regulations pointed out that the intention was 'to reflect a more positive approach to the use of residual hearing, and in this way to underline the importance of early diagnosis'.

By the 1944 Act education of the deaf became compulsory from five to sixteen, while education from two to five, and from sixteen to eighteen, became permissive. Local authorities were made responsible for finding out what children need special education, and to this end were authorized to examine them from the age of two. Spurred by the Ewings' work this led to the establishment of

* The Liverpool School for the Partially Deaf (1948), the Brighton School for the Partially Deaf (1949), Tewin Water School for the Partially Deaf (1953), Needwood School for the Partially Deaf (1954).

pre-school clinics and parent guidance programmes at Manchester University and at the Royal National Throat, Nose, and Ear Hospital in London, to audiology units like that at the Royal Berkshire Hospital in Reading, and to the provision of more and more special nursery schools or infant classes attached to existing schools (between 1947 and 1962 the number of deaf children under five attending such establishments was almost trebled).

Another development, made feasible by the improvement of classroom hearing-aids and by the free distribution of Medresco individual hearing-aids through the National Health Service since 1948, has been the opening of special classes or 'units' for partially hearing pupils in ordinary schools. The first four of these were set up in London in 1947. In 1950 a few deaf pupils were integrated experimentally into an ordinary school, Little Abbey School at Newbury (now removed to Liss in Hampshire), while a similar experiment began in the U.S. in 1954, when a group of selected pupils between eight and nine years old was transferred from a day-school for the deaf to an ordinary primary school in New York. In each case a specialist teacher of the deaf was attached to the staff of the school. But the idea did not begin to catch on until the 1960s, when the number of 'partial hearing units' attached to ordinary schools began to increase rapidly. By 1967 there were 189 such 'units' attached to ordinary primary and secondary schools, with a total attendance of 1,611 partially hearing pupils.* Graeser, in nineteenth-century Germany, had been the first to attempt to desegregate the deaf by attaching classes of deaf pupils to ordinary hearing schools; but the attempt failed because not enough allowance was made for the necessarily slower rate at which deaf pupils have to be taught. The revival of Graeser's ideal has been a postwar phenomenon in Britain and other countries, notably Denmark and the U.S., and owes a great deal to the development of the electronic hearing-aid. A trained teacher of the deaf is attached to the staff of an ordinary school, or a peripatetic teacher of the deaf visits several schools that have units of partially hearing pupils. He gives specialist teaching, advises the other staff about the problems of the partially hearing pupils, and keeps in touch with their parents. The system is not successful in all schools, but is undoubtedly one that offers much hope for the future. The handicapped pupils cannot always be

* See *Units for Partially-hearing Children* (H.M.S.O., 1967).

expected to do as well academically as their hearing companions, though many do. But the great advantage is that by learning and living with ordinary hearing children they are being better orientated and prepared for adult life in a hearing world.

Besides the growing number of these units, there are today more than seventy schools in Great Britain catering for well over 6,000 deaf and partially deaf children. For these schools there are over 800 qualified full-time teachers, trained either by the National College of Teachers of the Deaf, the Department of Education of the Deaf at Manchester University, or at the University of London, whose Institute of Education (Department of Child Development) now offers a course for teachers of the deaf.

This may be the place to glance at the state of the debate between the oral and silent methods, which continued to rage after the 'oralists' won their victory at the Conference of Milan. For most of the present century oral methods of instruction have been dominant, especially in Britain. But believers in the silent and combined systems fought a long and often bitter rearguard action against what they have sometimes come to refer to as 'the oral monopoly'. The argument has been a heated one, at times reminiscent of religious controversy.

The main case against the silent and combined systems is that finger-spelling or sign language marks the user off from the rest of the community and hinders him from integrating with it because he employs a different, and to most people incomprehensible, mode of communication. The signing deaf, as much as any minority group speaking a foreign language, tend to form an enclave separate from the bulk of the community. Indeed, some of the lay public (at least in Britain) look on signing and finger-spelling as a kind of witchcraft or at best an indication of mental impairment. Even professional deaf welfare officers seem inclined to treat the 'deaf and dumb' members of their clubs and missions as though they were children or incapable of unsupported responsibility for their own affairs. On this point Dr Pierre Gorman has noted in his unpublished thesis* that even when their deaf protégés can articulate and lipread, some welfare workers – to quote Dr Gorman – 'refrain from using oral modes which would otherwise lead to the development of a common or shared experience' because it might

* Pierre Gorman, *Certain Social and Psychological Difficulties facing the Deaf Person in the English Community* (1960).

lead to a 'reduction of superiority'. This is not intended to reflect upon welfare workers, who devotedly perform an exacting task and render an invaluable social service in a very difficult and neglected field, but to underline the way in which manual communication – even more than an unfashionable or ugly accent, for example – may bias people against its users. On the other hand finger-spelling and sign language, as no one can deny, are rapid and efficient media of communication, far more easily and successfully learnt and used than articulation and lipreading. For, sadly enough, the main case against the 'pure oral' system also rests on the isolation of the deaf person who has been educated by this means. Many of the congenitally deaf never learn to speak well enough to be easily intelligible to the average hearing person: indeed a Government Report published in 1968 indicated, disturbingly, that even today a substantial proportion of children leaving schools for the deaf are incomprehensible to all but their parents and teachers. Thus they find it difficult to integrate with the hearing world in any case; while so much time has been spent teaching them (more or less vainly) to articulate that they may have less command of language, and be less well educated generally, than if they had been taught by the silent or combined methods. Furthermore, as Dr Gorman has remarked in his thesis, there is the problem of the better-educated deaf person who feels an outsider in the deaf milieu yet is unable to fit in with the hearing community. It is the teachers of the deaf, rather than the deaf themselves, who have been most fanatical in the cause of 'pure oralism'.

Part of the bitterness of the dispute* has been due to the uncompromising stand taken by 'pure oralist' teachers against *any* form of signing whatever, from the finger alphabet to what may

---

* Its acrimony may be gauged from a now forgotten novel on the subject of deafness – *King Silence* by Arnold H. Payne, published in the first decades of the present century. Unlike so many novels dealing with deafness it is not guilty of sentimental falsification of the characters of its deaf protagonists (as is the case with even Carson McCullers's *The Heart is a Lonely Hunter*), though its documentary excellencies are spoiled by a novelettish plot. It is a spirited defence of the manual or silent systems of instruction and gives an illuminating picture of deaf education at the end of the nineteenth century in both England and America (the hero visits the U.S. to take a degree at Gallaudet College). Ann Denman's *A Silent Handicap* (1927) takes a more objective view of the oral–silent controversy and is worth reading, though written at a lower pressure.

fairly be called natural gesture. 'Pure oralists' insist on eliminating these aids because they tend to hinder the pupil's acquisition of articulate speech and to divert him from its use when acquired. On the other hand, two recent studies* would appear to discount this theory – though not wholly convincingly, according to the new Government Report on the education of deaf children.† The trend, however, seems to be towards a less militant attitude in respect to finger-spelling and signing. In Russian deaf schools, which were mostly oral up to 1950, it has become official policy to employ finger-spelling for the early teaching of language and speech, which in Russia begins at the age of three. The Danes have developed what is called the 'mouth–hand system' (sounds difficult to lipread are identified by the hand held to the mouth). In the U.S., where the deaf schools are now predominantly oral, a system known as the 'simultaneous method' is in use at Gallaudet College. This consists of the employment of all possible media – speech, lipreading, hearing-aids, signing and finger-spelling. And in Britain experiments are being conducted in at least two schools in the use of a new systematic sign language for the deaf, evolved by the late Sir Richard Paget.

As for the higher education of the deaf in Britain, I have already described the Mary Hare Grammar School. Most of its pupils take the General Certificate of Education examination at Ordinary Level, and quite a number of them continue to Advanced Level. Only pupils capable of profiting by a secondary education are accepted at the school: in 1968, 25 out of 126 candidates sitting for the entrance examination gained places. In spite of the advances I have detailed, it is depressing but perhaps salutary to have to quote the Principal's comment on these figures: 'Although this was the highest number of candidates to be entered it included a much larger proportion with very low academic attainments: at least forty were so poor that it is difficult to know why they were considered able to attempt a secondary education course at all.'‡ On the other hand the subsequent careers of Mary

* J. W. Birch and E. R. Stuckless, *The Relationship between Early Manual Communication and Late Achievement of the Deaf* (University of Pittsburgh, 1964). G. W. G. Montgomery, 'The Relationship of Oral Skills to Manual Communication in Profoundly Deaf Adolescents', *American Annals of the Deaf* (September 1966).

† *The Education of Deaf Children* (H.M.S.O., 1968).

‡ Mary Hare Grammar School Twenty-First Annual Report (1968).

Hare Grammar School ex-pupils have been encouraging. Every year three or four go on to universities, and many more to technical colleges, art schools, and the like; while others have become librarians, laboratory assistants and technicians, engineering draughtsmen, comptometer operators and programmers. Besides the Mary Hare Grammar School there are two others which offer secondary education for the deaf. Nutfield Priory School for the Deaf at Redhill, opened in 1949, provides a secondary modern curriculum for eighty pupils, while Burwood Park Secondary Technical School, opened in 1955, offers secondary education for thirty-five deaf boys.

All this is a long way from the sixteenth century when the education of the deaf was first seen to be possible; and from the eighteenth, when the first two schools for deaf pupils opened at Paris and Edinburgh. Nowadays, in the richer countries at any rate, much effort and money is spent on the education of the deaf, though the picture for the underdeveloped nations is of course far less happy.

The United States and the Scandinavian countries are among the most progressive and enterprising in dealing with the education of their deaf citizens and in helping the emergent nations to do the same. In America each state is in control of its own educational system, but in all states the education of deaf children is compulsory from the age of six and lasts for between eight and eleven years. There are three main types of school – state institutions, day-schools or classes, and denominational or private schools. While the many day-schools and private boarding-schools are purely oral, most of the state institutions teach by the oral method up to the elementary school stage, and after that give instruction by combined or simultaneous methods. In the field of vocational training the United States is paramount. Many large vocational schools for deaf children are lavishly equipped with advanced technical machinery provided free by local industries and business houses who value the services of well-trained deaf employees. At the Pennsylvania School for the Deaf nearly 200 different types and sub-types of vocational training are given: besides trades and skills like metalwork, printing, carpentry, needlework, hairdressing, automobile repair, building, plumbing, and so on, pupils are trained in every aspect of secretarial work – punch-card operating, comptometer-operating, and even the pre-programming of computer material. This particular aspect of the American scene typifies the healthier position of the American deaf adult who is more free to live an independent life with many more opportunities of employment than exist in Britain, despite the provisions of the Disabled Persons Employment Acts of 1944 and 1958 which requires businesses and industries to take on a quota of handicapped employees.

The American day-schools and private boarding-schools, like the famous Clarke School for the Deaf at Northampton, Massachusetts, are oral and most of them train their pupils for admission to high schools for hearing students – trade schools, business schools, art schools. Many go to ordinary universities, often via Gallaudet College or the big new Technical Institute (both of university status). Gallaudet is sponsored by the Federal Government and now has about 600 students, most from the state institutions and aided by a scholarship system. As Gallaudet provides teacher-training for both deaf and hearing students it has great influence on teaching methods in American deaf schools. Of these, counting state institutions, day-schools and classes, and denominational and private schools and classes, there was in 1963 a total of 452, catering for 30,577 pupils, of whom more than half attended the state institutions. Until fairly recently there was no separate education for partially deaf, or hard of hearing, pupils in America; either they were taught at deaf schools or they attended ordinary schools. Now this is no longer true, and many of the state schools – Pennsylvania for instance – have established partial hearing units attached to ordinary schools in their neighbourhoods. Many of the deaf schools have kindergartens for children under six, while nursery classes are often provided by local branches of the American Hearing Society, or by the audiology units maintained by many of the universities.

In France the educational system is more centralized than in Britain or the U.S. There are seven national and departmental institutions and thirty-two private or denominational institutions for the education of the deaf, all under the control of either the Ministry of Health or the Ministry of Education. Education of the deaf is compulsory and begins at six, though some institutions have kindergartens for younger children. After the age of fourteen pupils may go on vocational training courses, while the most gifted pupils may be selected to take advanced academic courses. There are four schools for partially deaf children, and as in the U.S. many of these children go to ordinary state schools, though there are no special classes provided. In the deaf schools the teaching is in theory mainly oral; the silent system of the Abbé de l'Épée ceased to be the official method of instruction in 1886. Audiology clinics are said to be held in the institutions and in some hospitals, where advice is given to the parents of deaf children, though a leading British audiologist who recently visited France came away with the impression that early diagnosis of deafness and parent guidance were so rare as to render oralism little more than an ideal rapidly degenerating into manualism, even for the partially-hearing children he met. And he found a surprising, and depressing, ignorance of international progress in the field of audiology.

Poland, East Germany, Czechoslovakia and Yugoslavia are further forward than France: one of the world's leading experts on early therapy is Guberina in Belgrade. He has developed the so-called 'Verbo-tonal method', a complicated cybernetic system for which he claims fantastic successes; but as they have proved difficult to duplicate his results have provoked some scepticism. In West Germany, the birthplace of 'pure oralism', there are now twenty-four state schools and eight private schools for the deaf. Compulsory education begins at seven, but some of the schools provide kindergartens. There are classes for partially deaf pupils in the ordinary schools of most big towns, but as these come under a different ministry there is not much contact between regular teachers of the deaf and those who teach the partially hearing. Most of the deaf schools offer compulsory continuation for pupils over the age of sixteen; they are usually vocational in nature, though one school at Dortmund offers a more academic type of education. In Holland there are three large residential schools for the deaf, including the famous one at Groningen which was founded in 1790 and the one in Gindhoven St Michaelsgestal which pioneered the use of music and dancing as an aid to improving the speech of profoundly deaf pupils. There are besides numerous small day-schools for partially deaf pupils. Education is compulsory from the age of seven, but there are many kindergarten classes and increasing provision of guidance for parents. Unlike West Germany, the state helps parents to pay for their children's hearing-aids.

In Denmark, the first country to make the education of the deaf compulsory, hearing-aids are provided free by the state. There are four state schools for the deaf, and in Copenhagen the State

Examination and Guidance Clinic for Deaf and Hard of Hearing Children gives audiological and psychological tests to infants and provides guidance for their parents. The four state schools are each equipped with an audiological laboratory in the charge of an audiologist. They are residential; but the Danes, like the Finns, have evolved a system which avoids congregating deaf children together as a separate community, by boarding the pupils out in foster-homes where possible. Besides the state schools, there are classes for partially deaf pupils attached to ordinary schools. Denmark was in fact the first country to separate deaf and partially hearing children for educational purposes. Teaching is oral, though in junior classes some use is made of Dr Forchammer's 'mouth–hand' system for lipreading, whereby some of the more difficult consonants are signalled while they are being pronounced. As for Norway and Sweden, education of the deaf has been compulsory since the eighties of the last century. Norway has four state schools for the deaf, two of them vocational, where trades are taught. One school, at Aln, provides a continuation course for brighter pupils. There are, however, only two kindergarten schools for deaf children under six, and both of these are privately financed. Sweden, however, has very many more, administered either by the state or by the municipalities, and is in advance of Norway in providing parent guidance at audiology clinics in Stockholm, Gothenburg and elsewhere. Hearing-aids are supplied free. Partially deaf children are taught in special classes attached to ordinary schools; for the profoundly deaf there are four state schools, at two of which vocational training is provided, while there is a continuation school at Stockholm for the academically gifted. In addition, the research centres into language growth and the new fields of psycho-acoustics are internationally famous.

But in the rest of the world, particularly in the newly independent countries of Africa and Asia, there are areas where the education of the deaf that exists is no more than a wave of the hand in the face of what needs to be done. Educating the deaf is a luxury in countries where much of the population is still illiterate and there are nothing like enough schools or teachers for the hale and sound. In such circumstances it is inevitably the handicapped who must be last served. Besides lack of resources, there are many other difficulties to combat, the multiplicity of languages and vernaculars, for instance. In Africa it is not unusual for a single tribe to speak literally dozens of dialects. There is even the problem –

from the lipreading point of view – raised by some languages like Chinese in which words are distinguished not by pronunciation but by differences in pitch or intonation. Nonetheless a great deal is being done, particularly by African mission schools in Kenya, Nigeria, Ghana, and Rhodesia. India, Pakistan, Ceylon and Malaya have their own schools. Many African and Asian countries send teachers to Britain and the U.S. for training; they on returning to their own countries are able to train more teachers locally. The problem is enormous, but no greater than that which faced the Abbé de l'Épée in the eighteenth century.

Afterword

FEW people know anything about deafness: why should they? Yet in spite or because of advances in medicine, deafness – like the population of the world – is on the increase. But so are techniques of combating and alleviating the disability. My own deafness came like a bolt from the blue; to begin with, my parents had no idea what to do about me or what might be done. This is usually the case with people who, nearly always unexpectedly, find themselves suddenly responsible for a child that has lost or may never have had its hearing. When I wrote this book I had my parents in mind, and people in their predicament.

Also I felt it would be a waste of opportunity not to attempt a report on the nature of the experience. Not much has been written about deafness by the deaf.* Even so, considering that I did not

* But see Molly Sefton's *Autobiography*, included in *Opportunity and the Deaf Child* by A. R. and A. W. G. Ewing (University of London Press, 1945) and Frances Warfield's *There's No Need to Shout* (Gollancz, 1949). There is Joachim du Bellay's *Hymne à la Surdité*, but I find it a rather banal counting of the blessings – or are they the *blessures*? – of deafness. Nonetheless, let me underwrite the following lines from the poem, which I here translate. The *Hymne* was addressed to Pierre de Ronsard, who lost his hearing as a result of being shipwrecked while escorting Mary Queen of Scots on her voyage from France to assume the throne of Scotland.

> All that I have of good, that in myself I value,
> Is to be without shame and without pretence, like you;
> To prove a good comrade, and to keep good faith,
> And to be, dear Ronsard, like you, half deaf:
> Half deaf! What a fortune! Would to God I had had
> Enough good luck to be deaf as an egg.
> I am not one of those whose inflated poetry
> Will create a mastodon out of a small fly,
> But without altering a white to a black colour,
> Or pretending a happiness to hide a dolour,
> I will say that to be deaf – for those who know
> The difference between good and evil (they are few) –
> Is not an evil, only seems to be so.

Heinrich von Treitschke, a nineteenth-century German writer and historian, describes his loss of hearing as a child in a poem called *Kranken-*

become deaf till *after* I had learned the language, I am no better placed than a hearing person to imagine what it is like to be born into silence and reach the age of reason without acquiring a vehicle for thought and communication. Merely to try gives weight to the tremendous opening of St John's Gospel: In the beginning was the Word. How does one formulate concepts in such a condition? 'Like watching a silent film without captions' is how one of the deaf-born recalled it. Still, the only way I can describe the experience of deafness is by drawing on my own; the first section of this book is, therefore, autobiographic. I was particularly careful to avoid reading about deafness while writing it. I did not want my own percepts and reactions to be influenced or diluted by other people's theories and observations. Once I had finished the autobiographic part I turned to the literature on deafness. Most of this I found on the shelves of the library of the Royal National Institute for the Deaf in Gower Street.* This literature is much larger than one would suppose; my heart almost failed me when first I surveyed the cohorts of books and journals there collected. Though I concentrated on the relatively few works containing information about the history of deaf education, I read a great many of the books on deafness and the deaf – all of them by non-deaf specialists – and ended up feeling considerably deafer than when I started. A minimal but frequent condescension of attitude and tone left me with a slightly depressed ego. Had I written the autobiographic portion of this book before instead of after I undertook this reading, it would have been a different account – perhaps less brash.

---

träume. Some extracts are quoted by K. W. Hodgson in *The Deaf and Their Problems*, but having no German I can't comment on them. The most accurate imaginative portrayal of what it's like to be deaf – though of one aspect only, its frustrations – that I have come across is Tristan Corbière's magnificent poem, *Rapsodie du Sourd*. It offers no false consolations, no pity or self-pity. One might also note that in the seventh book of Wordsworth's *Excursion* there is a portrait of a deaf man; but it carries no particular insights, though one cannot help admiring the

> tall pine-tree, whose composing sound
> Was wasted on the good Man's living ear.

* The R.N.I.D., besides being a centre of information and advice, maintains one of the world's largest and best libraries of books and periodicals concerned with deafness and allied subjects. I take this opportunity of expressing my gratitude to its librarian and library staff for their kindness and efficiency.

Nevertheless, in trying to project the experience of deafness autobiographically, it seems to me that I have unintentionally falsified the record so far as concerns myself. At one end of the scale there was a recent autobiography by a blind writer that barely mentioned his blindness – a gambit I can sympathize with – though it left one reader with a feeling of unreality and even disappointment. On the other hand the autobiographic sketch with which I have begun this book seems to go to the other extreme. In concentrating on those aspects of my life which deafness affected – after all, deafness is what the book is about – it is made to play a more prominent part in my existence than has actually been the case. The autobiography is selective; I would have had to write a much longer book in order to strike a balance. There are other defects. I have attempted no portrait of that remarkable woman, my mother, or of my father, to both of whom I owe even more than is implicit in this book.

The history of deafness, as I observed earlier, is the history of the education of the deaf. I have not been concerned with famous people who have had to combat the handicap, like Beethoven, Goya, and the inventor Thomas Edison, or lesser-known figures such as Harriet Martineau, Marie de Bashkirtseff, and Charles Maurras of *L'Action Française*. They make an odd bag; but in the case of some of them deafness occurred fairly late in life. It is after all only a few hundred years since the first attempts were made to rescue the deaf-born from their invisible intellectual dungeon by providing them with the keys of language. But now that the education of the deaf and technological developments in electronics are advancing hand in hand, intelligences that would otherwise be bound and gagged in languageless silence are being freed. This is one of the unequivocally valuable and encouraging aspects of progress in the present century.

Appendix

HEARING, DEAFNESS, AND RECENT RESEARCH
By K. P. Murphy, M.A., Ph.D.,
Deputy Director of the Audiology Research Unit,
Royal Berkshire Hospital, Reading

OF the five senses, hearing is probably the most precise. It is also probably the most complex. The senses are normally divided into two categories, those which detect events occurring outside the body and those detecting events impinging on the body. Touch and taste are concerned with the latter, whereas sight, hearing and smell, the so-called distance receptors, deal with the former. Sight deals with the light waves striking the body. Hearing deals with sound waves. Both these senses served to extend and enhance the sense of touch. My deaf friend can tell me that my car engine does not 'sound right' by resting his hands on the body of the car. My blind friend can tell me that it is a beautiful day because the sun's rays warm his face. But neither the deaf nor the blind person can detect sensations which occur at frequencies higher than the normal rate of transmission along the nerves: beyond that special organs are required. For instance, beyond 1400 cycles per second the touch or kinaesthetic senses require vision or hearing for specialized detection and discrimination.

Hearing is defined as the detection of sound by the ear and its transmission to the primary auditory area of the brain. In other words, the ear collects sounds and processes them in such a way that they can be dealt with by the particular part of the brain involved in auditory function. The range over which the healthy human ear can operate extends from approximately 15 to a maximum of 30,000 cycles per second. Animals hear even higher frequencies still, and in their case an additional skill permits focusing of the outer ear by lifting and turning it towards a sound. The experienced huntsman will watch his horse or dog because he knows that their ear movements will give him earlier warning and direct his own listening skills in the required direction. The outer ear has its visible and invisible parts. The visible part, the *auricle*, is embedded in the skull in the form of a long tube, which changes from fleshy to bony tissue and may be divided into three areas: meatus, middle ear and inner ear. Sound arrives in the auricle and travels down the meatus. Tightly stretched across the meatus a saucer-shaped membrane, the drum or *tympanum*, hides the middle ear, which in turn is separated from the inner ear by a bony wall. This bony wall is pierced by two small windows, one sealed with a tiny membrane of flexible tissue, the other with a small bony plunger. Because it is vibrating, the sound pulses upon the tympanum, setting it into vibrations, the resonance of which is determined by the sound pressures and the frequencies at which the sounds have reached the auricle. The middle ear, an air-filled cavity not much bigger than an orange pip, is also set into vibration through the tympanum and, being embedded in the skull, by the reverberance of the skull itself when sound strikes the head. This cavity is sealed at one end by the tympanum and at another by a bony wall, but there is a passage by which air reaches the middle ear. This is the *eustachian canal*, running from the front of the middle ear to the back of the nasal cavity in the throat very near to the adenoids. Air passing up this tube balances the air pressure applied by the atmosphere to the other side of the tympanum, so that if my ear drums have been affected by pressure changes after an air trip I can relieve the discomfort by pinching my nose and blowing it, thus pushing air back up my eustachian canals.

In the middle ear is a chain of three bones so tiny that the whole chain could fit quite neatly into the half moon on a well-manicured little finger nail. Yet the efficiency of movement of these three bones, the *malleus* (hammer), the *incus* (anvil) and the *stapes* (stirrup), can make a considerable difference to the efficiency of hearing. The vibrating tympanum moves the hammer which beats on the anvil which in turn causes the stirrup to rock. The stirrup is the bone which was earlier described as a plunger sealing one of the windows separating the middle from the inner ear. The third area, the inner ear, receives the sound in the main by this plunger and in part by the vibration of the part of the skull in which it is embedded. The inner ear is a sealed fluid-filled cavity, shaped like and about as big as a very small snail, and hence called the *cochlea*. This cavity lies within and towards the front of another fluid-filled cavity called the *labyrinth*. At the rear are the semi-circular canals which play an important part in bodily balance; thus certain disorders of hearing may be associated with dizziness or loss of balance.

If it were possible to unroll the cochlea it would be seen to consist of a coiled tube sealed at both ends and divided from end to end by a thin shelf composed of a bony ridge and a tough membrane. Imagine this tube filled with fluid and looking in cross-section rather like a flattened figure eight. At one end of the tube we see two windows. The first, in the upper half, is oval and fitted with a loose plunger, the stapes. The other, in the lower half, is round and sealed with a light membrane.

The tympanum, connected by its bony chain, transmits pressure to the upper sealed tube of fluid through the oval window. This pressure would burst the tube were it not allowed to escape via the thin shelf separating it from the lower tube. This, in turn, would also burst without some form of safety valve. Safety is achieved partly by the tube's own flexibility and partly by the action of the membrane sealing the round window. Here, then, is the ideal hydraulic system: pressure from the stapes causes the membraneous shelf or partition to bulge and ripple which causes the lower fluids to press against the flexible round window, and so the whole cycle is complete. Without the general flexibility of the tubes, the compressibility of the fluid and the round window to act as a kind of pressure valve the system, being sealed, could not operate and the middle membrane could not bulge and ripple. This last action is a vital part of hearing because the long membrane dividing the cochlea into our imaginary figure of eight supports hair cells called the *organ of Corti*. Sound, entering the ear by the relatively large meatus now concentrates its energy upon a much smaller aperture, the oval window. In turn this energy, converted by hydraulic pressure, sets the organ of Corti in motion and each hair cell may then become involved, as its turn arises, in a fantastic coding operation by means of which electrochemical changes in the nerve ends are initiated, and in an instant the electrical information passes to the auditory nerve joining the brain stem on its way to the auditory cortex. From start to finish the whole process has not taken longer than one three-hundredth of a second.

The description given above is necessarily incomplete, being designed as a simple illustration of one aspect of inner-ear function. Complicated as the anatomy may appear to be, the actual techniques of neural organization and transmission are so much more complicated that a number of theories have been advanced to help to explain them. There is a fairly general body of agreement about the major theories now, but their literature fills libraries (the reader wishing to pursue the topic will find that the library of the Royal National Institute for the Deaf is one of the foremost in this field in Europe, while in America he may use the Alexander Graham Bell Association for the Deaf at the Volta Bureau).

So far we have concentrated upon hearing. That is, we have taken sound energy and converted it to electrical energy arriving via the ear in the brain. What do we expect the brain to do about it? We know that one form of coding has occurred in the hair cells at the organ of Corti. Soon after this, another piece of coding has added information about directions and also set off a number of muscle movements. Maybe the head has swung towards or away from the sound. Perhaps breathing has stilled momentarily, the heart rate accelerated, the glands released adrenalin or, if the noise is startling in intensity or significance, set the limbs into reflex reaction – defence, flight, even collapse. At the same time other coding activities occur, demanding a complex physiological organization and initiating a state of greater or less attention. When the attention is engaged in auditory function and assists the brain in coding and decoding we talk of listening. No matter how good the hearing is, if the attention is not involved the person to whom the sounds are addressed may be quite unaware of them: they must attract his attention by making use of attention-provoking techniques. For instance, the man of the house, plunged in the evening paper, is unlikely to hear a request to put the kettle on, though he would hear an inquiry about his thirst delivered at the same sound pressure level. What is more, having heard the inquiry about his thirst, he would find difficulty in not hearing a request to put the kettle on if it followed the original question closely enough. Numerous experiments have shown that an infant will respond to his own name when ignoring other names from the same speaker at the same intensity. Listening is part of the intellectual and emotional organization of hearing and as such plays a most important part in auditory function. Because of this, factors modifying listening may lead to faulty diagnosis of the state of hearing. If such factors are persistent and extensive they can modify (or prevent) the development of speech in an infant. Perhaps it should be emphasized that modification of listening is not necessarily deliberate; in fact in the very young child this is rarely the case. Other sensory information may block auditory attention and in some other cases psychological or physiological factors may be the real cause, thus necessitating careful differential diagnosis and treatment.

Because it involves the brain, hearing is not a static thing; it is a skill which involves a complex psycho-physical process. As with any other skill, hearing matures with age, experience and the efficiency of the whole auditory process, mechanical, neurological, psychological, intellectual and emotional. In this sense hearing is vulnerable to any conditions which might modify any or all of these elements. The infant of five months, concentrating on visual stimuli, does not appear to hear: at least if he does hear he does not respond. However, if I reduce the light so that he cannot see, the same infant responds satisfactorily to auditory stimuli. The deeply disturbed child may not respond to sound unless specialized techniques are used. The adult deep in his book may not hear sounds unless they have certain special levels of significance. Certain types of brain damage may heighten the effects of auditory stimuli, others seem to reduce it. In the main, however, impaired hearing is most commonly associated with neuro-physical damage to the auditory pathways. These hearing impairments range from mild conditions to those of such severity as to be normally described as 'deafness'.

Deafness is usually conductive or perceptive in origin. 'Conductive hearing loss' refers to those conditions arising from some mechanical block in the transmission of sound in the ear. Causes range from such simple conditions as wax in the meatus, catarrhal fluid in the middle ear, or modifications of eustachian ventilation due to adenoids. Rather more severe conditions may be caused by immobilization of the bony chain due to dislocation or to fixation of the stapes in the oval window. The latter condition has yielded to surgery with increasing effectiveness in the last ten years or so. Investigation of the middle ear shows that bony formation (otosclerosis) has developed in the oval window, effectively 'silting up' the stapes and preventing the piston function already described. One of the most exciting events in the otological operating theatre is the patient exclaiming in jubilation when he hears once more during microscopic surgery under local anaesthetic.

Since the oval window measures only about one-twentieth of the area of the ear-drum the value of the microscope in surgery of this area is evident.

Perceptive (sensori-neural) deafness, as its name implies, results from some damage to the neural pathways between the inner ear and the brain. Investigation of the ear in patients deafened by German measles contracted by the mother in the early stages of her pregnancy show damage to the organ of Corti. Similarly meningitis damages the same organ and also the auditory nerve which connects the organ of Corti to the brain stem. At present nerve deafness cannot be helped by surgery; conductive deafness usually can and often is. Sometimes both conductive and perceptive deafness are present simultaneously, and the conductive element may be curable. This is important because many patients who have been told they have sensori-neural or perceptive losses purchase a hearing-aid and subsequently never consider the need for otological supervision. Clearly the patient wearing a hearing-aid still has a little hearing (or the aid would be useless). A developing conductive loss (commonly described as a conductive overlay) may so reduce the remaining hearing that the aid becomes increasingly useless. Hearing-aid wearers should never acquire a more powerful aid without first discovering whether or not their deterioration is conductive. A short visit to the otologist may result in considerable saving, financial and emotional. However, it should be said that visits to otologists are rarely productive of miracles; travelling from one surgeon to another in hope of a miracle cure wastes patients' and otologists' time. The patient who has been told that he has a sensori-neural loss, and that there is no conductive overlay, could save himself considerable disappointment by accepting this advice.

Hearing impairment may arise from inherited factors or from infections occurring before or after birth. It is most important to differentiate between hereditary causes and congenital causes. An infant born deaf may not have inherited the deafness, in fact the odds are quite high against it. This means that deaf persons whose deafness is due to pre- or post-natal infection need not fear that they are more likely to have deaf children. They might be more likely to have deaf children if they married another deaf person, but even there the likelihood is increased only if they marry somebody with inherited deafness. For this reason much of the research into deafness is aimed at identifying causes and recording them as early as possible in the life of the child. The most obvious reason for this is that infections during pregnancy often give rise to multiple damage, and the early care of the child, advice to parents and future education can be planned more accurately if the cause is known.

Since we are thinking of early diagnosis let us consider how early deafness can be diagnosed. Response to sound can be demonstrated before birth. Researches in half a dozen or so centres throughout the world are reporting increasingly accurate techniques of producing a brief spurt in the heart rate of the unborn infant by sound stimulation. Accuracy is maintained by preventing the mother from hearing the sounds, by checking that her own heart rate does not change, by checking that nothing happens in the uterus (sudden movement, small contractions of the abdominal wall, etc.). After this, a small telephone applied to the mother's abdomen feeds sound in and a small microphone similarly placed transmits the foetal heart sounds to an amplifier and recorder.

Though such results can be produced, it is far too soon to say that these methods will ever become a reliable test for deafness. The same comment applies to much of the work which is now in progress on the response to sound of the newly born. Not long ago I was able to demonstrate the response to sound of an infant aged fifteen minutes. The demonstration took place in Bombay in the course of a lecture and study tour: by a stroke of fortune, this infant, lying flat on her back with her head gently supported, flicked her head towards quiet sounds and screwed up her eyes and flicked her head away from louder sounds. However, the fact that some infants do respond does not mean that all will, nor that those who do not will not respond subsequently. The simplest elements of discomfort can cause an infant to ignore sound. Failure to respond needs extensive re-checking before a decision about deafness can be made. For all this, it is now possible to say with reasonable accuracy by four or five months of age that a child is or is not profoundly deaf. We cannot say that the child who responds will never be deaf nor can we say that the child who responds will always understand speech. Where, owing to the medical history of the mother or the infant, the risk of such conditions seems greater, we in England can arrange routine supervision as part of the National Health Service. Under this supervision, delayed speech or deterioration of response to sound can lead to further investigation and the initiation of the correct therapeutic procedure should they be required.

The main urgency for early diagnosis lies in the need to maintain infant vocalization. Perhaps it is not generally understood that the deaf infant is rarely mute. Muteness arising from deafness tends to occur later in infancy because the infant, failing to hear his own voice, soon loses interest in it. He ceases to play with his voice, bouncing it off the walls or off his family. He sees his family's delight, but cannot know that his early babbling is the cause, so voice begins to go. His mother grieves, deprived of a basic need in her relationship with the child. Long before the child is aware of his deafness he may well be aware of a change in his mother, tension, distress, fear, guilt. Meanwhile the developing skill in gesture is likely to become the true 'mother tongue'.

Diagnosis, then, leads to therapy, guidance for the mother, and instruction in the best approach to her problem. Ideally the six-month-old deaf infant will have started to wear a hearing-aid, his voice will be maintained as the foundation for the slow, laborious process of developing speech and language. Skill in using the remnants of hearing will begin to grow.

These days there is a wide range of facilities for deaf education. A secondary grammar school is complemented by a secondary technical and several secondary modern schools. There are boarding-schools and day-schools for deaf children and also for those with partial hearing. In addition, over the last decade, a new development has occurred – the establishment of the Partial Hearing Unit and the service of travelling teachers of the deaf (now officially described as peripatetic teachers). By means of these two services, large numbers of deaf children are educated close to home within their local community and attend special classes attached to ordinary schools. Many of these classes send their children into the main school for assembly, play, meals and non-academic pursuits, since the aim is to keep these children in close contact with their hearing neighbours. Induction loops fastened throughout the school and arranged around the playground allow the child with a hearing impairment to be within reach of amplification. Though some quite profoundly deaf children may well manage in such systems the units are, of course, more successful with partially hearing children.

The peripatetic teacher is employed to help the child wearing a hearing-aid in an ordinary school to make the best possible progress. Although the figures are published annually I am often surprised how few of my colleagues know that there are practically as many children wearing hearing-aids in ordinary schools as there are children being specially educated because of faulty hearing. Last year, of approximately 12,000 school-children diagnosed with impaired hearing, nearly 5,000 were wearing hearing-aids in ordinary schools.

The social results of such changes are likely to be considerable; the educational results are already being felt. Some of the traditional residential schools for profoundly deaf children are beginning to complain of the large numbers of deaf children in their schools with additional handicaps. Some attempt to meet their need is being made with schools for children with more than one defect: blindness and hearing impairment, cerebral palsy and hearing impairment, deafness and emotional disturbance, deafness and intellectual retardation, are all provided for to a certain extent. The melancholy fact remains that increased skill in saving infant life is creating an increased number of damaged babies who will make heavy demands on the educational services.

What can we expect in the future? Probably there will be a considerable reduction in the incidence of congenital and adventitious deafness (the hearing impairment arising from trauma or infection). Hereditary deafness is unlikely to decrease significantly for many years to come, while the increased skill in maintaining life already mentioned will produce a further temporary crop of problems. At present we expect about two children of every thousand to be born with a hearing impairment. Slightly fewer than half of these will be profoundly deaf, probably the same proportion will be congenital, and will contain all types of hearing loss. Very mild degrees of hearing impairment occur much more widely than is commonly known. Scandinavian research indicates that one child in ten can expect some hearing problem during school life. Although outside the scope of this book, mild hearing loss seems worth mentioning particularly because of its likely psychological and educational consequences. Research on educational retardation and reading problems has inculpated quite mild hearing disorders. Hearing losses which would not be noticed in the front of the class cause severe modification of listening skill in the back rows. Some authorities insist that every educationally retarded child should have a hearing check.

Another factor which we tend to ignore is the danger of damage to hearing arising from loud noises. Such defects as 'boiler-maker's deafness' have been known for a long time, but what of tractor-driver's deafness, firing range deafness, aircraft deafness, taxi-driver's deafness? All these conditions are appearing with increasing regularity in the professional literature and there is no doubt that in the years to come more claims will be made against employers for their alleged failure to protect workers against noise. A recent paper given to an Audiological Conference showed that prolonged exposure to loud pop music in enclosed conditions can cause temporary modification of hearing. Because temporary modification has been alleged to lead to permanent damage of hearing after prolonged exposure to sound, this particular phenomenon will no doubt be studied with considerable care. As well as causing hearing impairment, noise causes stress, leading to fatigue and error. Humanitarian considerations apart, since inefficiency, stress and error cost money, industrial designers should concentrate on minimizing the effects of noise.

David Wright has alluded to the apparent equability of the deaf person. Perhaps one day this will be properly investigated. Should it be established one element might well prove to be freedom from noise-induced stress. Patients recovering from severe illnesses are often irritated by noise; the next decade or two could see the development of special soundproof recovery areas in hospitals. Sometimes I long for just one room in my own house which is as quiet as that in which I carry out my research. I don't want to be deaf (though as the years roll on I do not expect to maintain perfect hearing) but I have now exchanged my childhood fantasies of a 'cap of darkness' for a 'cap of silence' to be assumed or left off at will. How many school-teachers long for the same thing? Simple expedients like reducing echo in corridors, assembly halls, and stairways have been shown to cut down school-children's own tendency to make noise. When finance permits it, one expects that schools will be designed in such a way that study areas are protected from noise. All the same my most enduring memory of school is the lazy sound of the mower on the cricket pitch, the click of a bat on ball and the somnolent bird song drifting in through the open windows. Perhaps as time goes on we may combine the best of both worlds – good, silent conditions for study and the flick of a switch to provide enough background noise to keep us awake!

For the profoundly deaf child, research is now moving with

increased rapidity. Nearly thirty American Universities have major projects into problems of deafness. In England shortage of funds has slowed the pace, but even so the recently established British Society of Audiology has shown that a tremendous amount of work is going on here. Scandinavian countries have exciting machines in hand. New devices for attempting to make use of the remnants of hearing are being designed; new ways of training the ear are being investigated in Yugoslavia; new methods of visual display will be studied in the University of Sussex in the next few years. It is true that the deaf adult would probably not want hearing after prolonged experience of deafness, but I am sure he would not wish to deprive the deaf child of the best we can give him. Similarly the adult faced with sudden deafness or the insidious impairments of old age will pin his hopes to the successful outcome of current research. Nevertheless, curing profound deafness is not yet within sight. For many generations to come, profoundly deaf children will need all the support they can get; so will their families and the communities in which they work. It is here that I see one serious problem. Machines may help the deaf child a little, but building machines seems to be easier than changing attitudes. Until society realizes the unlocked potential in the deaf child, both the child and society will be the poorer. For all our efforts to detect and deal with deafness, for all our improved educational facilities, our care for the deaf adolescent entering employment, for the deaf adult needing social or psychiatric care, is frighteningly inadequate. We have much to learn from the Italians, the Americans, the Swedes and the Danes in these areas, but fortunately the omens are good; social workers are increasing in number, psychiatric provision is just beginning, some employers are beginning to cooperate. But whatever the improvements the person deaf from birth will need all his courage, his skills, his sense of humour, his patience and persistence. Above all he will need language skills. The fact that one or two highly intelligent deaf men have achieved great things, have even managed to become poets, should not blind us to the intellectual starvation of the rest.